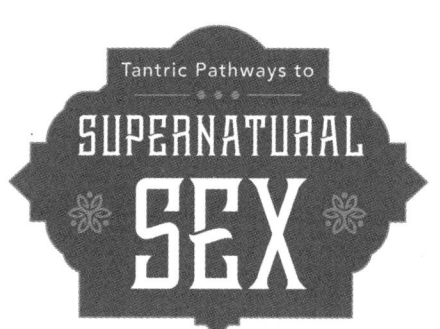

Tantric Pathways to
SUPERNATURAL SEX

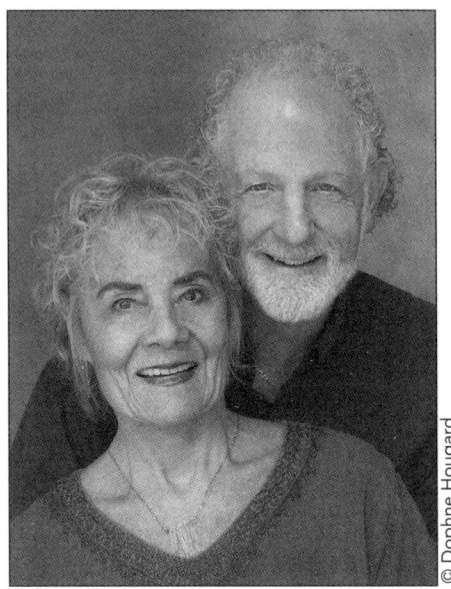

About the Authors

Jeffre TallTrees, PhD

Jeffre is an author, workshop leader, experienced executive, and licensed psychologist with over thirty years of clinical experience specializing in relationships, human sexuality, and energy medicine. After earning a BS in nursing from UCLA, she served as a labor and delivery hospital nurse, a public health nurse, and a mental health nurse for Los Angeles Country. Jeffre received her PhD from the California School of Professional Psychology in 1977. She was continuing education and volunteer director for The Open Door drug abuse prevention project for four years. She founded a holistic health center in North Hollywood in 1977 and was program director for Cambia Way, an intermediate mental care facility, for three years. From 1980 through 1982 she was director of the Family Stress Center in Concord, California, and became active in local politics and agency funding. During that time, she was chairman of the Human Services Advisory Commission of Contra Costa County. She was acting director of mental health for Tuolumne County in 1982.

She was in private psychology practice from 1981 until 2005, specializing in marital and sexual therapy as president of Danville Psychology Associates. With a colleague, she coauthored *Intimacy: A Green Light For Red Hot Sex*, which was published in 1997. For ten years in the '80s and '90s, Dr. TallTrees wrote a weekly psychology advice column titled "Let's Talk" for four local newspapers in Contra Costa County, California. After years of membership, she became president of the Bay Area Clinical Hypnosis Society in 1994 and ran monthly meetings and conferences. Jeffre was a longtime member of AASECT, the American Association Of Sexuality Educators, Counselors, and Therapists, and presented at its 1997 and 1998 national conventions.

After studying with Margot Anand in 1996, she completed her sacred sexuality teacher training and served as an instructor for her year-long Love And Ecstasy Training from 1995 to 1998. She also completed the series of six Sex, Love, And Intimacy workshops hosted by the Human Awareness Institute. As cofounder of Tantra At Tahoe since 1998, she teaches workshops and counsels clients on conscious sexuality. Jeffre has coauthored three books on intimacy and Tantric sex. In 2001 Jeffre received her certification as a massage practitioner from the School of Shiatsu And Massage at Harbin Hot Springs, California. Jeffre presented the latest sexuality breakthroughs at the national Lifestyles Convention in Reno and Las Vegas 2002, 2003, and 2004. After completing his Light Body School in 2005, she served as lead teacher for Dr. Alberto Villoldo's Four Winds Society, an international academy of shamanic energy medicine until 2011. In 2009 she founded SacredRainbowMesa.com through which she sees private clients and teaches energy medicine workshops. She has spoken publicly many times, been interviewed on local TV, and been quoted in newspapers. She even appeared briefly on CNN while meeting Barack Obama during his first presidential campaign. Jeffre's latest presentation was to the Women Empowering Women conference in California during 2016.

Jeffre is a shaman, healer, counselor, workshop leader, artist, football fan, and avid skier living near Lake Tahoe, California with her husband Somraj and their two spaniels, Sage and Pixie.

Somraj Pokras

Somraj is an entrepreneur, published author, website designer, workshop leader, public speaker, and counselor. He received a BS in organic chemistry from the California Institute of Technology in 1968. During his master's program at the University of Southern California, he served as assistant director of the IntraScience Foundation and coordinated its first two international cancer chemotherapy conferences. He began his speaking career in 1971 by giving monthly talks for a community counseling center he cofounded with fellow students in West Los Angeles. His first of many keynote addresses was in Malmö, Sweden, in 1972, where he had the rapt audience of over two hundred in stitches. He received an advanced certificate in interpersonal counseling in 1972 from the Advanced Organization of Copenhagen. In 1973 he served there as technical director overseeing all training and counseling before moving to their Los Angeles academy in 1974, where he was senior case supervisor for the counseling clinic.

He learned to apply the social expertise gained during his counseling career to the business world by teaching for New York–based Effective Communication Skills Inc. from 1975 to 1977. He presented Effective Presentation Skills workshops to Bankers Trust Company, Bank of America, Wells Fargo Bank, and the FCB, Foote Cone & Belding, advertising agency.

Somraj's next career centered around the Viability Group Inc., the management training consultancy he founded in 1974, where he managed a team of consultants, trainers, and support staff. During his thirty-year career as a management consultant, he developed and presented public speaking, presentation, interviewing, management, and time management skills workshops for Bank Of America and multiple University Of California extensions. He served as training director for the Bank of California during 1976. As a keynote speaker and workshop leader for Fortune 500 companies, government departments, and public agencies around the world, Somraj designed over fifty workshops that guided over twenty thousand people to lead more effective lives. That included Skills and Tact In Dealing With People for IBM in San Jose, Palo Alto, Atlanta, New York, Tampa, Montreal, Amsterdam, and Stockholm. He wrote and taught the Systematic Problem-Solving and Decision-Making workshop for Chevron for many years which was published by Crisp Publications in 1989.

In the 1980s he presented Managing Staff for Results workshops at major universities nationwide to nonprofit executives through the Public Management Institute. During this time, he developed his unique format of how-to training guides for Viability Group's twelve core people skills programs. Over the years he designed, wrote, and published dozens of custom editions for clients. He has spoken at conferences and taught for other firms such as Westinghouse and Siemens plus government departments like the Social Security Administration, the California State Compensation Insurance Fund, the Farm Credit Administration's Production Credit Associations, and POST, the Peace

Officers Standards & Training agency. He presented Public Relations and Fundraising workshops for the Public Management Institute. Somraj has taught expert witnesses from the California Public Utilities Commission how to testify in court and handle cross-examination.

He served as president of the Silicon Valley Chapter of the American Society For Training And Development in 1988. During his tenure he ran monthly professional meetings with hundreds of participants, led association conferences, and gave keynote addresses. In 1989 he designed, wrote, and conducted the week-long Team Leaders And Facilitators Bootcamp for the Council For Continuous Improvement and its member companies, including Motorola and National Semiconductor. Later he conducted train-the-trainers programs and turned nine of his trainings into print books, including *Rapid Team Deployment* and *Working In Teams*. He also designed a custom Effective Listening Skills program for Intel.

Somraj entered the sexuality field in 1997 by studying with the internationally acclaimed sexologist Margot Anand. After graduating, he served as an instructor for her year-long Love And Ecstasy Training from 1997 to 1998. He also completed the series of six Sex, Love, And Intimacy workshops hosted by the Human Awareness Institute. With his wife, Jeffre, he cofounded Tantra At Tahoe in 1998, where he teaches workshops, counsels couples, and continues to write its monthly Sacred Sexual Secrets newsletter. Along with his partner, he's written ten ebooks about Tantric sex and has a successful fifteen-year track record selling ebooks to over one hundred countries through the website he designed and maintains. In 2001 Somraj received his certification as a massage practitioner from the School Of Shiatsu And Massage at Harbin Hot Springs, California. He presented the latest sexuality breakthroughs at the national Lifestyles Convention in Reno and Las Vegas 2002, 2003, and 2004. He received his certification as an energy healer through Dr. Alberto Villoldo's Light Body School in 2007.

Somraj derives great joy from assisting others in releasing sexual inhibitions that block their pleasure so they can thoroughly enjoy all parts of life and love. He is a certified bodyworker, private pilot, avid skier, rock hound, mountain biker, passionate music lover, football fan, and skilled lover. He lives near Lake Tahoe, California with Jeffre and their two spaniels.

Praise for *Tantric Pathways to Supernatural Sex*

"*Tantric Pathways to Supernatural Sex* has everything any lover needs who wants to harness the dormant powers of their libido and sex drive. In simple steps, it suggests ways to make sexual intercourse more loving, more electric, and more orgasmic. Its 'supernatural' angle shows how to catapult all kinds of erotic encounters beyond the ordinary. This down-to-earth lovemaking manual is easy and fun to read solo or together for men, women, and same-sex partners of all ages and experience."

—Caroline Muir, author of *Tantra: The Art of Conscious Loving* and *Tantra Goddess: A Memoir of Sexual Awakening*

Jeffre TallTrees and Somraj Pokras have written a book based upon their years of study and research into what makes a truly fulfilling sexual relationship. With their new book they join the ranks of important contributors to the evolution of human sexuality. I highly recommend this book."

—Johanina Wikoff, PhD, psychotherapist and author of *The Complete Idiot's Guide to the Kama Sutra*

"*Tantric Pathways to Supernatural Sex* uses yogic breathing, movement, and sensibilities to enhance sexual pleasure. And if you're not into yoga, the book provides a welcome introduction to *kundalini*, the ancient Indian term for sexual energy, and guides you through new and exciting ways to think about making love."

—Michael Castleman, author of *Great Sex* and the *All About Sex* blog for *Psychology Today*

"From the very first page, *Tantric Pathways to Supernatural Sex* by Jeffre TallTrees, PhD, and Somraj Pokras speaks to exactly what you want to experience sexually with your partner. It encompasses all the essential ingredients that generate passionate lovemaking, including chemistry, energy, and electricity. It offers user-friendly techniques to harness them in a way that will promote extraordinary sex. It is a must-read for those who are looking to bring vitality and a reenergized sense of life to their intimate time together, so as to take their shared pleasure to a new horizon."

—Dr. Jane Greer, New York–based marriage and sex therapist and author of *What About Me? Stop Selfishness from Ruining Your Relationship*

"Jeffre and Somraj take us into the most intimate moments of sexual union to show us that ecstasy is the most blissful path to the Divine. Let these two masters who have tasted the infinite lead you to discover new realms of intimacy, love, and enlightenment!"

—Alberto Villoldo, PhD, bestselling author of *One Spirit Medicine* and *Shaman, Healer, Sage*

"Somraj and Jeffre capture their combined forty-six years of experience in Tantric practices with elegance and fun. They have revised classic techniques to match their personal style and present information clearly. Their depth of knowledge and understanding of the lineage allows the reader to quickly understand this beautiful practice with clarity."

—Nisi & Thor, founders of Tahoe Tantra

"When you read this book, I am certain that you will recognize the experience that happens every time you enter into your den of love. It's magic, mystical, and supernatural."

—Joy Day, CEO of Joy Day Wellness

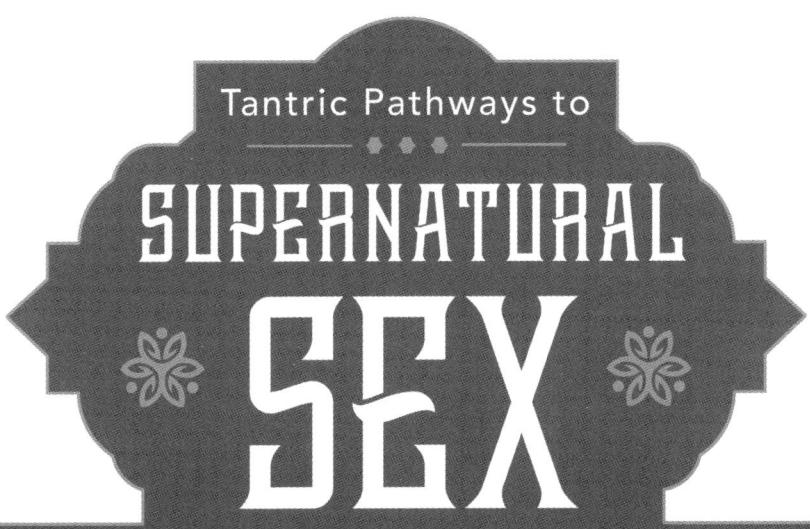

Llewellyn Publications
Woodbury, Minnesota

Tantric Pathways to Supernatural Sex: A Groundbreaking Look at the Chemistry of Sexual Electricity © 2019 by Somraj Pokras and Jeffre TallTrees, PhD. All rights reserved. No part of this book may be used or reproduced in any manner whatsoever, including internet usage, without written permission from Llewellyn Publications, except in the case of brief quotations embodied in critical articles and reviews.

FIRST EDITION
First Printing, 2019

Cover design by Kevin R. Brown
Interior illustrations by Mary Ann Zapalac

Llewellyn Publications is a registered trademark of Llewellyn Worldwide Ltd.

Library of Congress Cataloging-in-Publication Data
Names: Pokras, Somraj, author. | Talltrees, Jeffre, author.
Title: Tantric pathways to supernatural sex : a groundbreaking look at the chemistry of sexual electricity / Somraj Pokras & Jeffre TallTrees, Ph.D.
Description: First edition. | Woodbury, MN : Llewellyn Publications, [2019] | Includes bibliographical references and index.
Identifiers: LCCN 2019013414 (print) | LCCN 2019015689 (ebook) | ISBN 9780738760315 (ebook) | ISBN 9780738760230 (alk. paper)
Subjects: LCSH: Sex instruction. | Sex—Religious aspects—Tantrism. | Sexual excitement. | Sexual intercourse.
Classification: LCC HQ31 (ebook) | LCC HQ31 .P757 2019 (print) | DDC 613.9071—dc23
LC record available at https://lccn.loc.gov/2019013414

Llewellyn Worldwide Ltd. does not participate in, endorse, or have any authority or responsibility concerning private business transactions between our authors and the public.

All mail addressed to the author is forwarded but the publisher cannot, unless specifically instructed by the author, give out an address or phone number.

Any internet references contained in this work are current at publication time, but the publisher cannot guarantee that a specific location will continue to be maintained. Please refer to the publisher's website for links to authors' websites and other sources.

Llewellyn Publications
A Division of Llewellyn Worldwide Ltd.
2143 Wooddale Drive
Woodbury, MN 55125-2989
www.llewellyn.com

Printed in the United States of America

Other Books by Somraj Pokras and Jeffre TallTrees, PhD

Print only
Intimacy: A Green Light for Red Hot Sex and a Lifetime of Loving

Print and Ebook
Male Multiple Orgasm: Techniques That Guarantee You and Your Lover Intense Sexual Pleasure AGAIN and AGAIN and AGAIN

Female Ejaculation: Unleash the Ultimate G-Spot Orgasm

Ebook only
Ultimate Premature Ejaculation Mastery: The Ecstatic Solution to Unlimited Sexual Stamina

208 Kama Sutra Tantra Sex Positions: The Complete Illustrated Guide to the Ancient Love Guide's Postures

Supreme Bliss Tantra Guide to the Ecstasy of Spiritual Sex

Tantric G-Spot Orgasm & Female Ejaculation: Awakening Her Sacred Gate to Supreme Bliss

Tantric Male Multiple G-Spot Orgasm: Awakening His Sacred Gate to Supreme Bliss

Hotter Sex, Deeper Love: A Couple's Guide to Ultimate Intimacy

*We dedicate this book to all the lovers throughout our lives
who've helped us evolve in and out of bed.*

*And to the Tantra teachers who brought this wisdom to the modern world
and inspired us to reach for all we could be.*

And to each other for our undying passion and eternal love.

Contents

Exercises xv
Authors' Note xix
Introduction 1

PART 1: The Pathways... 9
Chapter 1: Supernatural Sex   11
Chapter 2: Energy Tools   17
Chapter 3: The Tantric Attitude   25
Chapter 4: Partnering   35

PART 2: Loveplay and Sweet Spots (Phase 1)... 43
Chapter 5: Loveplay   45
Chapter 6: Vajra (Penis) Anatomy   53
Chapter 7: Yoni (Vulva & Vagina) Anatomy   59

PART 3: Kundalini... 71
Chapter 8: Energy   73
Chapter 9: Channels   79
Chapter 10: The Five Cornerstones of Ecstasy   87

PART 4: Penetration and Initial Entry (Phase 2)... 99
Chapter 11: Initial Entry   101
Chapter 12: Sexual Positions   109
Chapter 13: Rosetta (Anal) Sex   125
Chapter 14: Energetic Clearing   137

PART 5: The Valley (Phase 3)... 143
Chapter 15: Settling into the Valley   145
Chapter 16: Strokes and Schemes   151
Chapter 17: Power and Balance   159

PART 6: Kundalini Currents ... 171
Chapter 18: Channeling Ecstasy   173
Chapter 19: Flowing Sexual Electricity   183
Chapter 20: Energy Linkages   191
Chapter 21: Peaking and Plateauing   201

PART 7: Climbing (Phase 4) ... 211
Chapter 22: Physical Orgasms   213
Chapter 23: Energy Orgasms   223
Chapter 24: In Orbit   229

PART 8: Closing (Phase 5) ... 237
Chapter 25: Savoring the Closing   239

Conclusion   243
Contact Us   245
Bibliography   247
Index   251

Exercises

Chapter 3
Conscious Breathing   26
Corpse Posture   27
Body Honoring   28
Last Stroke Technique   29
Heart Meditation   30
Self-Pleasuring   31

Chapter 4
Partnering Questions Discussion   38
Communication Tools   40
Sacred Space   41

Chapter 5
Tantric Touch   47
Loveplay   48

Chapter 6
Exploring Vajra   58

Chapter 7
Exploring Outer Yoni   62
Exploring Inner Yoni   67
Yoni Erection   70

Chapter 8
Pleasure Balloon   77

Chapter 9
Chakra Breathing   82
Inner Flute   85

Chapter 10
Presence   89
Tantric Breath   89
Love Sounds   90
Erotic Movement   91
Find Your Pelvic Floor Muscles   93
Kegels   94
Visualization   95
Orgasmic Breathing   96

Chapter 11
Initial Entry Discussion   104
Vajra Yoni-Massage   104
Initial Entry   107
Soft Entry   107

Chapter 12
Sexual Postures   120
Yoni Sweet Spots   122

Chapter 13
Gradual Insertion Method   130
Rosetta Entry   134

Chapter 14
Yoni Clearing   139
Rosetta Clearing   141

Chapter 15
Dancing on the Verge   148

Chapter 16
Strokes and Schemes   154
Slow Variety   156

Whimsy   156
Short Cycles   157

Chapter 17
Receiving   162
Synchronizing   166
The Shiva-Shakti Game   167

Chapter 18
Feeling Kundalini   175
De-armoring   176
Releasing Blockages   177
Running Energy   179
Raising Kundalini   180

Chapter 19
Voltage   185
Loosening Your Body   187
Streaming   188

Chapter 20
Hot Links   195
Connecting Passion Circuits   197
Connecting Energy Circles   198

Chapter 21
Solo Peaking   203
Surfing Peaks   205
Partner Peaking   207
Solo Plateauing   208

Chapter 22
Male Orgasm   215
Female Orgasm   218
Other Orgasms   220

Chapter 23
Implosive Orgasm   226
Full-Body Orgasm   227

Chapter 24
Extended Orgasms   231
The O-Zone   232

Authors' Note

Neither the authors nor the publisher are engaged in rendering medical or any other professional service. The educational practices and sexual techniques described in this book should not be used as an alternative to professional medical treatment, psychological counseling, psychotherapy, or any other services best performed by a health professional. This book does not attempt to give medical diagnosis, treatment, prescriptions, or suggestions for medication in relation to any human disease, pain, injury, deformity, or physical or mental condition.

Absolutely no part of the program should cause pain or unusual symptoms. It is recommended that you consult your physician to obtain a diagnosis for any physical or mental symptoms you may experience.

If you have knowledge or suspicion that you have contracted a sexually transmitted disease, we urge you to consult with a qualified health professional before engaging in any partner practices described in this book.

The authors and publisher of this book are not responsible for any upsetting reaction, divorce, damage, injury, infection, fatal disease, or other adverse outcome as a result of applying the information or engaging in any activities suggested in this book.

The stories shared in this book are based on real-life events and experiences. Many of the names and some of the circumstances have been changed to preserve privacy.

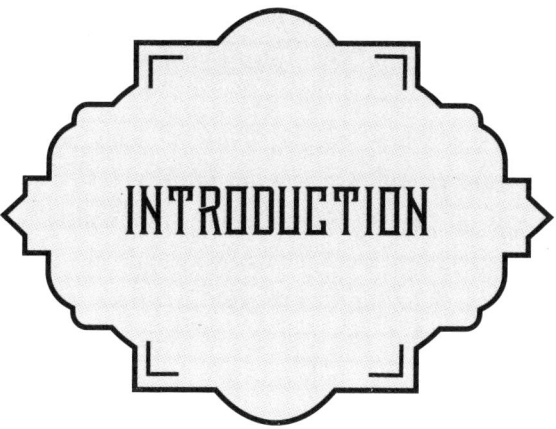

INTRODUCTION

We live at the mercy of our passions. The spiritual lifeforce energy that runs through all of us fuels these emotions.

Have you found that love and sex bring the most joy and wreak the most havoc in your life? Few of us are in conscious control of sexual energy, or what the ancients called *kundalini*. Our Tantric path has shown us how to become the master of these passions, thereby enriching our lives.

Without kundalini rising, you wouldn't get turned-on, feel pleasure, reach orgasm, or be launched up to that divine altered state that peak lovemaking offers.

There are primal forces inside that few lovers ever befriend. Sure, there's the physics of friction from kisses, licks, touches, strokes, and thrusts. But the metaphysics of making love—consciousness, emotion, spirit, energy—really determine whether or not you reach passion, orgasm, fulfillment, and sensual ecstasy together.

It's kundalini that excites your body. It makes your nerves fire, breath deepen, skin flush, and muscles twitch. The electrical currents streaming and the fire sparking inside create both subtle and intense sensations. You've felt them move, right?

Connecting hearts, exchanging kundalini, and merging spirits with All That Is is what makes sex sacred.

Pathways

Tantric Pathways to Supernatural Sex explains how you can develop the style of lovemaking that we call Supernatural Sex.

Supernatural Sex is a kind of sexual union that's beyond ordinary sex. Though it's extraordinary and may seem mystical at first, it's not really magic. It doesn't just focus on orgasm but creates a continuously orgasmic state of shared passion. You might even call it a pathway to divine communion.

This holistic approach to Tantric sex expands intimacy and sensuality by activating multiple heart, mind, and soul connections while you give and receive pleasure.

Tantra began as a powerful grassroots shamanic practice in India thousands of years ago. It's more about mindfulness, meditation, and enlightenment than sex. Tantric exercises can heighten spiritual consciousness, body awareness, and, as a result, the flow of kundalini or sexual energy.

Like other ancient Eastern philosophies, Tantra is a path to enlightenment. But in contrast to most religions, Tantra is about the total union of sex and spirit.

Tantric Pathways to Supernatural Sex shows you how to activate both ends of the spectrum—spiritual connection and orgasmic sex—at the same time. It shows you how to focus your mind to stimulate your body. It explains how to revel in physical pleasure to elicit a spiritual response from your tissues. And connect your sacred nature with your beloved while making love.

This Book

Tantric Pathways to Supernatural Sex is a how-to guide about transforming your love life into everything you've ever dreamed of. Like other erotic guides, it covers desire, anatomy, erogenous zones, foreplay, intercourse, peak pleasure, and orgasm.

But unlike others, its theme is the role of sexual energy, the spiritual force that fuels your life. This book is a groundbreaking look at the chemistry of sexual electricity: how bodies couple, hearts blend, emotions react, minds interact, and souls merge.

Even though parts of this book may be familiar, there's a lot that will be startlingly new to you. Even eye-opening.

Here you can get your burning questions answered about this sexual lifeforce. Where is it? How can you free it? What activates and supercharges it? How can you channel it? How does it help you grow spiritually? How can you exchange it with your beloved? What makes it erupt into cosmic fireworks?

Is *Tantric Pathways to Supernatural Sex* for you? Yes, if you want more in your sex life. Yes, regardless of your age, gender, lifestyle, or relationship status. Yes, if you want more intimacy, more passion, more orgasms, and more connection with the Divine.

This book is for

- adventuresome lovers who want to go for everything,
- long-term couples who've lost the zest in their sex life,
- LGBTQIA lovers who want to fully harness their dormant kundalini,
- new partners who find they aren't clicking so well in bed,
- younger lovers who want to understand anatomy and arousal, and
- older lovers with waning libidos.

After reading and practicing, you'll have more sex because you'll want it more often. Supernatural Sex will make you feel more alive, more vibrant, more healthy, and more peaceful. When your sexual encounters leave you feeling energized and empowered, you'll easily want to make more time for it.

Supernatural Sex

Since we're guessing that, like the rest of us, you weren't issued an operating manual for your sex life, most of the sex you've had is probably on the ordinary side of the spectrum.

Supernatural means beyond natural, beyond the ordinary. Why is Supernatural Sex extraordinary? Because it helps you feel each other's passion and get consumed with the ecstasy of love. Because it lets you embrace the universal lifeforce energy surging through and between you. And because it transports you to a state of extended orgasm.

Ordinary sex can be fun. But to connect hearts, merge souls, and play at the edge of the mystical is a whole different story. When you learn to tap into the otherworldly powers of sex, you might deem it supernatural. If you can already easily soar with the Divine through sexual play, we applaud you. The rest of us mere mortals need education and training to get there.

Tantric Pathways to Supernatural Sex teaches you how to use sex in a way that fulfills your soul's deepest needs for connection with your lover and with the Divine. It offers pathways to touch the Divine every time you touch each other to share pleasure.

We know that sex is sacred and the desire for sex is sacred. We believe it is the most beautiful and rewarding act you can give yourself and your relationship.

To get there, you charge yourselves and each other with erotic electricity. You generate ongoing waves of pleasure that get stronger and stronger the longer you do it. Instead of a quick eruption, you feel like you're coming all over, over and over, for as long as you want.

Although Supernatural Sex isn't magic, harnessing your innate erotic charge and becoming continuously orgasmic can launch you to an altered state that feels magical. We'll open the door to a whole range of startling new passions we call energy orgasms. Then, kundalini pulses through your body, extending out to reach your partner, letting the two of you vibrate all over with fiery sensations and feel the ultimate intimacy.

In Supernatural Sex, the physical sexual act becomes a spiritual meditation. Your mind quiets, your body relaxes, and you melt into the fabric of space-time together, only wanting more and more forever.

This merger of your physical energy with the spiritual energy of the universe will galvanize you to dance in the sky together for as long as you want.

Our Approach

We began studying Tantra in the 1990s and it's our continuing practice that has transformed ordinary sex into Supernatural Sex.

We—Jeffre and Somraj—are two mature, experienced professionals and a long-term married couple. Jeffre began her career as a PhD sex therapist twenty-five years ago when few other female psychologists practiced this specialty. Though trained as an organic chemist, Somraj spent thirty years as a Fortune 500 people-skills training consultant.

Tantric Pathways to Supernatural Sex is written like a candid conversation between trusted friends. It focuses on the real stuff that happens to you in and out of bed.

We draw on everything from our decades of study starting with the latest discoveries of modern sexology. That's interweaved with the lost lore of ancient mystics from India, Arabia, and China and the energy healing practices of indigenous shamanism.

We hope you're not squeamish about frank talk because we confront all the glorious details of sexual pleasure and sexual intercourse. Bluntly, but tastefully. And relate some hot stories to make our points.

We wish more lovers talked about sex like the poets of the Ming Dynasty in China who called the act of love "clouds and rain." Regretfully, there are too many dirty words for making love. We prefer nontechnical, nonprofane language that reflects our sacred view of love.

You'll encounter a few special terms like *jewels* for genitals and *jewel union* for sexual intercourse. Instead of penis we prefer the Tantric term *vajra*. And we use the Sanskrit word *yoni* in the place of vulva and vagina.

You'll also see us using interchangeable terms for different levels of arousal, turn-on, and excitement roughly arranged in order of intensity: sensation, pleasure, chemistry, erotic charge, sexual electricity, erection, passion, orgasm, and ecstasy.

No worries. We promise to define anything new and remind you occasionally.

Responsible Pleasure

This how-to manual empowers all lovers to be fully responsible for their own pleasure regardless of their gender, lifestyle, or sexual preferences.

That means whether you're male or female, young or old, single or coupled, gay or straight. To make the language simpler, you'll find us using *he* and *she*, *male* and *female*, instead of every conceivable pronoun. When it's important, we'll refer to the *giver* and the *receiver* of pleasure, which doesn't depend on gender.

Though we have a decidedly sex-positive attitude, it's not our goal to disturb or shock you. Still, we should warn you that some of our forthright anecdotes and explicit suggestions may stretch your comfort zone.

You have the choice to skip what falls outside your comfort zone and move on. Just recognize that you can stay where it's comfortable or consciously choose to explore, practice, and even risk a little like we have.

Tantric Pathways to Supernatural Sex guides you to approach the subject of sacred sex as a research team of two spiritually aware beings studying how to expand sexual pleasure. Ultimately, you can't do this unless you're willing to experiment.

Our nonjudgmental approach is designed to make it safe and easy for you to try new things. We'll show you how to put a toe in water instead of jumping in blindly.

Still, we don't assume that you'll try or like everything we've attempted.

Our job is to relate what's worked for us and others. We just hope you'll be open-minded about our progressive advice. It's up to you to determine what works for you and for your relationship.

Five Phases of Sexual Response

William H. Masters and Virginia E. Johnson pioneered research into the nature of human sexual response with their groundbreaking studies starting in 1957 at Washington University in St. Louis. They recorded some of the first laboratory data on sexual anatomy and physiology by direct observation of women and men making love in the laboratory.

Notably, Masters and Johnson clearly defined the four stages of the body's response to physical stimulation: *excitement* (initial arousal), *plateau* (full arousal short of orgasm), *orgasm,* and *resolution* (post orgasm). They observed that most lovers' arousal levels out or plateaus after initial excitement. That causes them to push for more and more pleasure, resulting in an explosive orgasm.

Supernatural Sex follows a similar sequence of five phases:

1. Loveplay (part of *excitement*)
2. Initial Entry (part of *excitement*)
3. The Valley (the *plateau*)
4. Climbing (*orgasm*)
5. Closing (*resolution*)

We've broken the excitement stage into *loveplay*, or what most lovers call foreplay, and *initial entry*, or first penetration. This is because lovers who practice Supernatural Sex may revert to talking, touching, and oral sex (usually reserved for foreplay) anytime during coupling. And because initial entry is such a critical step in penetrative sex, especially for women.

We call Masters and Johnson's plateau stage the *Valley* because it's a safe, warm place where arousal levels out. It's a place you want to stay and play in. A focus of Supernatural Sex is to extend the Valley as long as possible before climbing to orgasm in the fourth, or climbing, phase.

Their resolution stage refers mostly to physiology, so we've renamed it *closing* to identify loving and intimate things essential after lovemaking.

This Book's Eight Parts

Tantric Pathways to Supernatural Sex is organized into eight parts, with a few chapters within each part.

PART 1, The Pathways, defines the overall journey and its foundations.

PART 2 is about Sweet Spots and Loveplay (phase 1). These chapters are about arousal, getting turned-on, and stimulating *sweet spots*, our name for erogenous zones.

PART 3 is Kundalini, the Eastern name for sexual and orgasmic energy. Here we introduce underappreciated methods of harnessing and channeling your dormant sexual lifeforce to give you access to a whole new universe of pleasure. You might call it sexual ecstasy.

PART 4 is entitled Penetration and Initial Entry (phase 2). Here we'll dive into jewel union (sexual intercourse), including first penetration, sexual positions, anal penetration, and energetic healing.

PART 5 is about the Valley, which is phase 3. Here is the central focus of Supernatural Sex, namely extending your pleasure by creating stroking patterns that result in sweet rhythms. The chapter about balancing power is vital to create a partnership dedicated to lasting ecstasy.

PART 6 is Kundalini Currents. In these chapters we'll show you how to direct the flows of kundalini by connecting hot links, opening passion circuits, connecting electrical circuits, merging energy fields, and exchanging orgasmic energy. These two parts about the Valley conclude with a vital chapter about peaking, or how to surf intense peaks of sexual pleasure.

PART 7 is about Climbing to orgasm, which is phase 4. Climbing begins when your peaks are so intense that you're ready to go for it. We cover multiple ways to climax singly and together both physically and energetically. It concludes with climbing beyond the ordinary toward different kinds and higher levels of orgasms that we refer to as *in orbit*.

PART 8, Savoring the Closing (phase 5), is about how to enjoy the afterglow of the energy you've shared in an intimate and loving way.

After laying the foundations of Supernatural Sex in PART 1, PART 2 will give you a detailed review of a man's twenty and a woman's thirty erogenous zones or sweet spots. Starting in PART 3 we'll show you how to find and excite them to release kundalini or sexual energy. In PARTS 4 and 5 we examine the mechanics, dynamics, and energetics of jewel union (sexual intercourse) like no other book does. PART 4 is about initial penetration and PART 5 addresses extending your pleasure in what we call the *Valley*.

PART 6 explains how to open your energy channels and flood yourself with passion. This includes hooking those channels up with your beloved. Then you can stay in the Valley as long as you want and transform your coupling into a continuous orgasmic flight.

It all comes together in PART 7, which covers the whole spectrum of both physical and Tantric energy orgasms. PART 8 deals with phase 5, which is the closing.

Now that we've introduced the aims and structure of *Tantric Pathways to Supernatural Sex*, let's get started with PART 1.

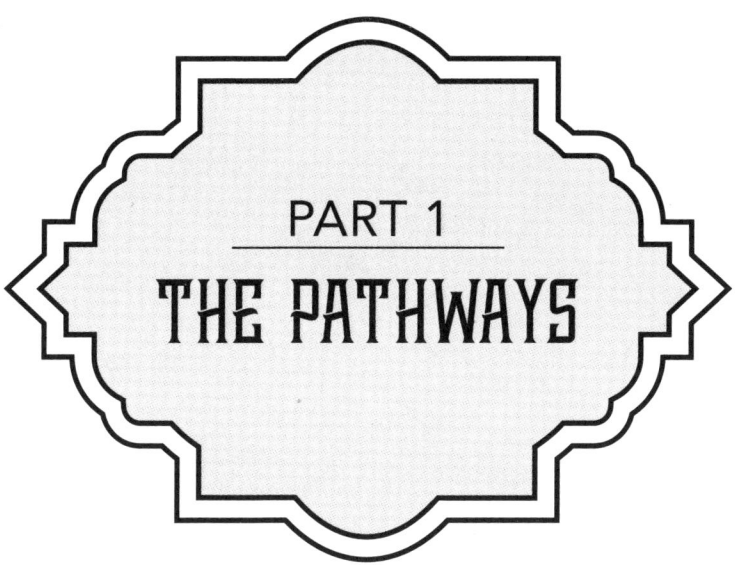

PART 1
THE PATHWAYS

PART 1 gives the helicopter view of the Tantric pathways to Supernatural Sex. We explain what that really means in chapter 1. In chapter 2, we give you an overview of sexual energy tools that come later. Then we'll share how to build a solid platform for the whole journey in chapter 3 using the Tantric attitude. Chapter 4 is about partnering.

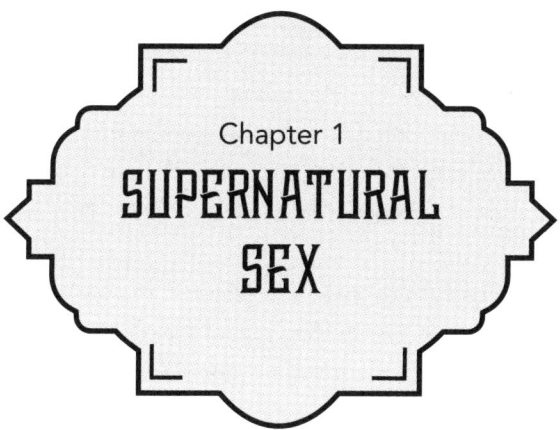

Chapter 1
SUPERNATURAL SEX

Our pathway to Supernatural Sex really began when, in our fifties, we met at a spiritual sex workshop in 1996. The irresistible sexual chemistry that swept us away made our first encounters super exciting.

We thought we were pretty good at it. When we started practicing Tantra together, we discovered how much more there was. Now we know that Supernatural Sex doesn't just happen. You have to grow it together.

In this chapter we will paint a picture of where this book is going. We hope you'll use it to create a vision of the kind of sex life you want.

Ordinary Sex

To us, ordinary sex is a biological process ruled by lust and regulated by hormones. Quick release and fast orgasm are its goals. That's where we started. It was great when we both got there on occasion but frustrating when we didn't.

Ordinary sex can look like a movie scene where two strangers rip each other's clothes off in a wild frenzy and do it on the floor or against the wall. More like a sport, the contestants rush toward maximum turn-on until exploding in a blaze of glory.

Or, with long-term partners, ordinary sex goes through the motions like nobody's home. Or the guy with so much pent-up lust convinces his partner to do things she wouldn't otherwise consent to.

Sure, sometimes ordinary sex feels good. But it usually amounts to quickies. Studies show that the average time for sex is five to ten minutes. Regardless of what she gets, most men roll over and fall asleep after coming. On the other hand, Supernatural Sex can last for hours if you want.

When we were first together, our ordinary sex usually resulted in an *orgasm gap*. That's the well-documented fact that men come more often than women. On occasion, though, one or both of us reached a remarkable height of passion. At first, we didn't understand how we got there. That didn't allow us to repeat it at will.

We weren't guiding each other so our pleasure was hit and miss. There was more nonstop jack-hammering and less regard for each other's energy.

In short, we weren't making love on multiple levels of body, heart, mind, and soul at the same time.

Tantra

Studying and practicing Tantra allowed us to transform ordinary sex into Supernatural Sex.

Tantra is an ancient Eastern spiritual philosophy based on the metaphysics of sexual energy. It teaches how to raise consciousness and harness the life-forces inside that drive sexual desire and everything else. Because Tantric practices combine sexual and spiritual energy, it's often referred to as spiritual sex or sacred sexuality.

The first Tantra teachings emerged in India some seven thousand years ago as a grassroots rebellion against the repressive hierarchical religions of the day. Tantra sprang up as a movement to make spiritual illumination and ascension available to all, not just to the privileged castes via a priest or shaman.

Early Tantra writings described practices, meditations, and secret rituals that prescribed a path to liberation and enlightenment. These esoteric Hindu texts were a dialogue between the archetypal male god Shiva and the archetypal female, his consort Shakti.

That's a basic concept of Tantra that was later echoed by the psychoanalyst Carl Jung. We both have masculine and feminine energies within that need to be unified.

Tantra showed us how to accept and love all of who we are so we could open fully to our divine nature. That allowed us to experience more pleasure, bask in extended ecstasy, and regularly catapult each other to peaks higher than ever before.

The *Kama Sutra* and More

We often reference the *Kama Sutra*, the Hindu love manual that depicted the sexual customs of upper-class Indians about fifteen hundred years ago. That made it much different than the spiritual Tantric writings.

The *Kama Sutra* was totally forthright about things many people are too ashamed or embarrassed to talk about. Things like seduction, foreplay, jewel (genital) sizes, sex toys, aphrodisiacs, and sexual postures. Maybe that's why it's so popular today.

We also draw on erotic literature from Egypt and Arabia, such as the fifteenth-century Arabic sex manual *The Perfumed Garden of Sensual Delight*, written by Muhammad ibn Muhammad al-Nafzawi.

We've received sexual guidance from Taoist masters from ancient China as well. Taoism is a Chinese philosophy based on the writings of Lao-tzu from the sixth century BC. Central to Taoism is inner contemplation and mystical union with nature, which explains its similarity to Tantra. Taoist sexuality began as a branch of Chinese medicine devoted primarily to longevity.

Supernatural Sex

There are many ways to make love: cuddles, quickies, or longies that are sweet, slow, or rough.

Supernatural Sex is the style we prefer, one that connects us at multiple levels. It's a conscious approach to harnessing and sharing sexual energy. By consciousness we mean acute awareness of your sensations and desires creating a holistic sense of where you and your partner are at all times.

This is an intimate, loving, partnered way of connecting in which you communicate more before, during, and after. Sometimes it's slower so you can savor intense pleasure. And sometimes it's wilder as you discover new peaks, climaxes, and altered states.

Making love this way is more like meditation than athletics. That's because your mind isn't busy plotting and planning, judging and justifying, wondering and worrying.

Supernatural Sex isn't a scripted performance. It's a joining together in a spontaneous, easy, yet mindful way.

During Supernatural Sex you will experience continuous waves of pleasure that stream through you. It's focused on building an intense boil of passion that lasts longer and becomes stronger than any quick physical release.

Aren't you interested in experiencing all the luscious feelings of ecstasy and orgasm but for much longer than the typical ten-second release?

Supernatural Sex uses your lifeforce to connect your hearts, merge your souls, and release waves of sexual electricity all around you and between you.

There's an innate magnetic intelligence in the body that few lovers take full advantage of. Most are so busy thinking or fumbling around they don't get out of their own way and let their uninhibited nature take its course. They don't allow their erotic electromagnetism and dormant bio-energies to engulf them.

To get there, you have to really grasp sexual anatomy and technique. But the real secret lies in consciously harnessing sexual energy by accessing the inner reservoirs of untapped power that lie dormant within. That's how you can reach such intense and prolonged levels of ecstasy.

An Example

To give you an example of Supernatural Sex, we want to share with you a particularly moving erotic encounter.

Even though we were so hot for each other that we wanted to rip each other's clothes off, we silently bowed and touched foreheads. We looked into each other's eyes, breathed together in meditation, and shared our desires and concerns.

As we undressed each other ritually and whispered sweet endearments, the heat sparking between our bodies rose to a fever pitch. The first slow, subtle caresses were like the discharges of a powerful electrical storm. Our nerves reacted as if hit by lightning.

Our hands explored everywhere and were magically drawn by that irresistible magnetism to our hard and wet spots. Our ping-ponging moans shook the rafters. Each time we nearly exploded from the torrent of pent-up sexual energy, we purposely slowed. With a moment of silence and a few deep breaths, we surrendered to the spasms reverberating inside.

Penetration, when we couldn't resist any longer, was like being transported to a different realm. The intense sensations were more like an inner hurricane than a warm summer's breeze. To savor every last drop of pleasure, we moved at a snail's pace at first. Then one of us sped up, then the other thrust deeper, then the first relaxed into the incandescent heat.

Fast, slow, deep, shallow, pausing, side to side, up and down, our motions smoothly shifted in a kaleidoscopic rhythm of colors and hues.

Finally, we understood how scientists harness nuclear power, letting the radiation in the reactor build very gradually to create a steady flow of electricity instead of the detonation of an atomic bomb.

Ever so slowly, the delightful in-and-out strokes created wave after wave of tingling excitement, rush after rush of pulsing heat, and spasm after spasm of cellular vibrations. After each peak of pleasure, we relaxed to let the energy wash through and between us.

We were in no hurry, with no place to go, simply absorbing every last calorie of delicious sensation we could glean from each motion.

As our bodies merged with less and less separation, pulsing one inside the other, the peaks rose higher and higher. We seemed to contain so much sexual energy that an explosive orgasm would have blown our heads off. But no matter how our animal selves craved release, our higher selves didn't want to end the ascent.

On and on we rode each other, sometimes fast, sometimes slow. Positions morphed, electricity sparked between us, and one's tremblings became the other's quaking. Time seemed to stop as the distance between us melted away. What one of us felt, the other felt. We vibrated as one, joined in divine union.

Though we wanted to go on forever, our bodies eventually needed fresh air, water, and sustenance. Locked on each other's eyes, we knew it was time.

Without so much as a change in our rocking rhythm, the vibration in our groins simultaneously began to grow. It was as if an electromagnetic fist embraced our jewels and pulsed deep into our flesh. Sparks arced up, down, and around as our bodies filled with liquid fire, surging with ecstasy.

We felt each other teetering on the precipice. Surrendering to the irresistible force, the vast, dark, empty void reached up to embrace us. All we could do was relax and go with the flow. Floating for an instant that seemed to stretch out for ages, we gave ourselves—body and soul—to the infinite power of the universe.

Mother Earth and Father Sky shot bolts of lightning through our bodies. We were falling and soaring at the same time.

Convinced we couldn't ascend any higher, the first jewel spasms hit us both at the same instant. Spurting like a tidal wave and clenching like an earthquake, we began to come together. We screamed, laughed, cried, and howled, outdoing each other's loudness.

Each successive convulsion seemed stronger than the last and threw our bodies to and fro across the soaked sheets. We reveled in the sounds, smells, and sensations of our wet work of art.

At last the fist of the Divine stopped shaking us and we collapsed in each other's arms moaning "Oh My Goddess!" over and over.

Partnership

As our story shows, Supernatural Sex is a lovemaking partnership in which you connect as equals and share power. This intentional union of minds and bodies begins by connecting as spiritual beings. That starts with knowing yourself, sharing what you want, and exercising your power.

Being naked this way in front of each other means more than just shedding your clothes. For most lovers this requires a new attitude, a fresh way of thinking, and a different way of approaching each other. Respect, patience, listening, and consideration are crucial.

Because whoever is receiving pleasure knows what's best in each moment, you want to exchange leading and following. Instead of the guy performing and the gal hoping he does a good job, you collaborate. Sometimes one of you focuses on giving while the other is receiving pleasure. And then you swap roles.

Lovers in Supernatural Sex are much more animated than in ordinary sex. Receivers clearly show their passion and givers willingly respond. The receiver often leads by asking, signaling, responding, and guiding.

Summary and Action Steps

- Honestly consider what your sex life is like currently.
- What would you like it to be ideally?
- Share these thoughts with your partner. If your playmate isn't interested, you may find it helpful to journal your thoughts and reactions from here on.
- If you can, agree on reading this book together and doing its exercises.

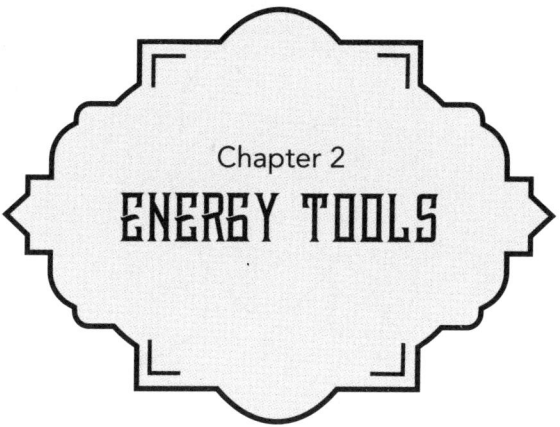

Chapter 2
ENERGY TOOLS

To master Supernatural Sex you need to be able to feel, harness, and direct sexual energy. Chapter 2 is an overview of the tools you'll see later on.

When you're getting sexually turned-on, you can feel a small trickle of nervous stimulation and physical excitation, alive, bubbling, moving, and vibrating inside you. This is sexual energy, which you probably feel most strongly right before and right after orgasm.

Sexual energy is the electromagnetic lifeforce in the human body responsible for attraction, sexual desire, libido, sex drive, turn-on, pleasure, and orgasm. We call it sexual energy when it charges your pleasure centers, and orgasmic energy when it makes you explode over the top.

The old Sanskrit name for this normally latent psychosexual power is *kundalini*. The kundalini is pictured as a coiled snake lying dormant at the base of the spine as shown in figure 1, Kundalini at Rest, on page 18. When awakened through Tantric, yogic, erotic practice with or without sexual play, kundalini can ascend through your subtle energy body, the bio-energetic field or *biofield* that surrounds you. You can feel it as pleasure and passion that make you vibrate, shiver, and shake all over.

Although kundalini is always there, sometimes it's quiet. When sleeping, its sensations are subtle. You'll see this kind of energy referred to as subtle energy. It's like a higher, finer frequency that's hard to hear until you're turned-on and tuned-in.

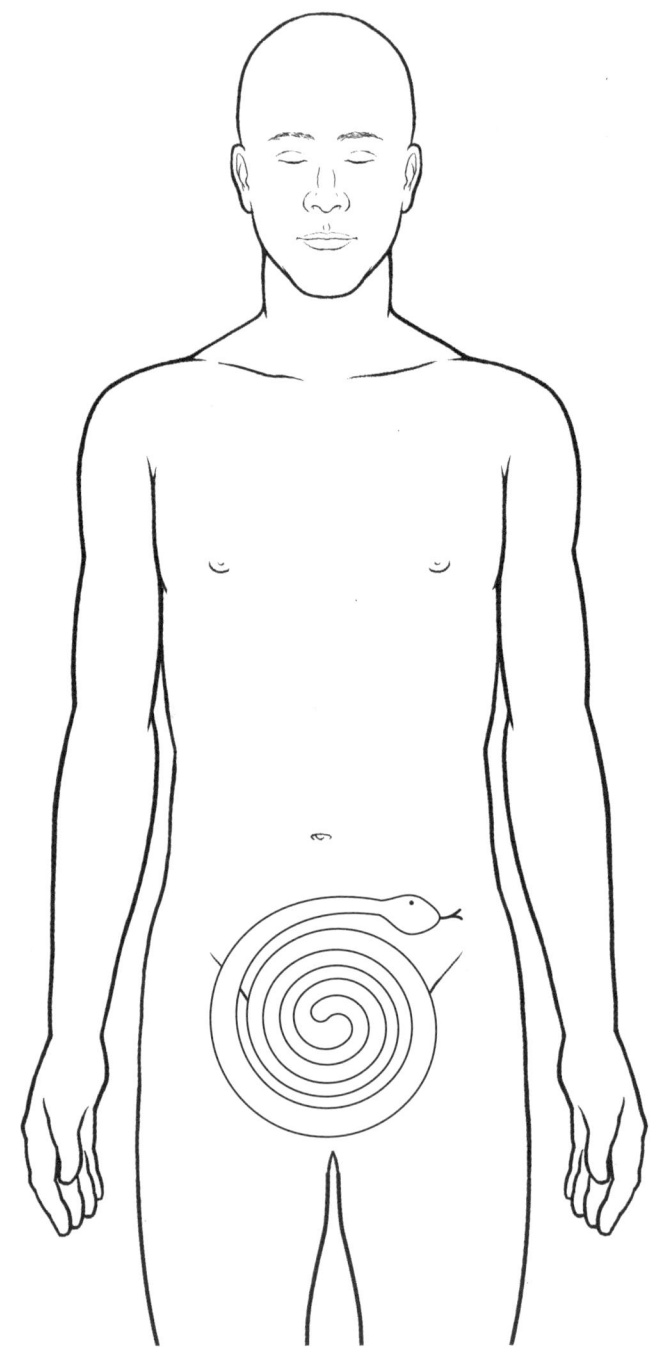

Figure 1: Kundalini at Rest

When awakened, kundalini becomes a potent power that you can feel flowing inside you. Then this subtle energy becomes a tidal wave of lifeforce that can dramatically move you.

Kundalini streaming through you can create a state of ecstasy, an almost overwhelming state of euphoria, rapture, and bliss. Sometimes it awakens a heightened state of cosmic consciousness.

Sweet Spots

There are many more inner fountains of kundalini, typically referred to as *erogenous zones*, than most people know how to access.

In fact, there are twenty erogenous zones in and around a man's jewels (genitals) and thirty in and around a woman's. We're not just referring to the clitoris and G-spot but many more inside and out.

We call these particularly sensitive tissues *sweet spots*. If you've ever hit a tennis ball perfectly right and felt that powerful zing, you know what we mean. Exciting your own or your beloved's sweet spots is what produces blossoms of pleasure.

In addition, pooling kundalini can awaken sweet spots other places in the body. Have you ever found sexual electricity sizzling in your hands, feet, back, head, or unidentified zones inside? When charged, you can boost your pleasure by playing with these energetic sweet spots.

It's these kundalini flows that make your nerves fire, your tissues vibrate, and your screams erupt. A primary aim of Supernatural Sex is to target your sweet spots to amass as much kundalini as you can hold and make the ecstatic state last.

Mastering kundalini gives you access to Tantric *energy orgasms*. That's where you enjoy all the delightful sensations of physical climax without releasing much of your energy. Which makes it possible to come again and again and again.

In this continually orgasmic state, there's a lot going on inside your body. The fireworks produce all sorts of waves, rays, and streamers, plus pulses, surges, and currents, that all result from the electromagnetic vibrations that spread and settle in different tissues.

Needless to say, to get there requires more than just reading this book. It requires dedicated practice.

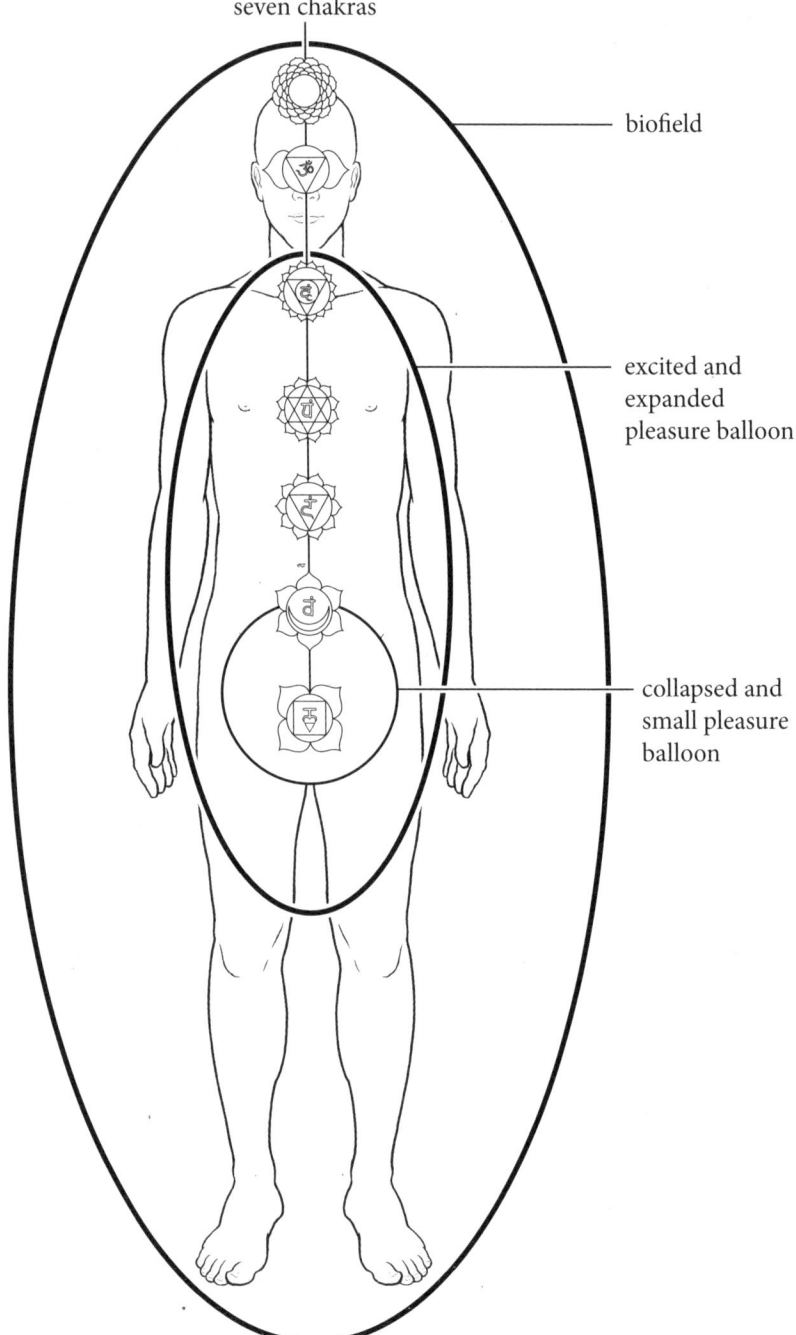

Figure 2: Pleasure Balloon

Pleasure Balloon

When energy moves inside, it creates a field that some call your energy body. When electrical impulses travel through your nervous system or kundalini pulses between various subtle nodes, these currents create a magnetic field. In other words, the more turned-on you are, the stronger this biofield becomes.

We've found it helpful to visualize a *pleasure balloon* inside the body. That's an imaginary bubble filled with kundalini. At rest, the small balloon is collapsed around your jewels as shown in figure 2, Pleasure Balloon, on page 20.

As you get excited and pump it full of energy, it expands to ultimately fill your entire biofield. The bigger your pleasure balloon, the more delicious sensations you feel in more places.

This energy field is intimately interconnected with your *chakras*. The chakras, from the Indian word for wheels, are seven energy centers arrayed from the bottom of your pelvis to the top of your head. They govern your rainbow of lifeforces, human magnetism, and different types of body electricity in all the ways that kundalini manifests.

Peaking

Have you ever found yourself falling into a really yummy groove while making love? We call those times when you never want it to stop *sweet rhythms*. You can learn a lot about creating sweet rhythms from sex positions and thrusting patterns from the *Kama Sutra*, Taoists, and modern sexology.

Hitting sweet spots pumps kundalini into your pleasure balloon. Too much too fast can pop it, triggering an explosive orgasm before you're both ready.

Knowing how to back off at the edge of coming, or what we call the skill of *peaking*, is vital in Supernatural Sex. When you can dance on the verge of orgasm over and over, you'll be able to make those erotic peaks higher and higher and last longer and longer.

Eventually peaks of pleasure merge into plateaus of ecstasy. When your body is clear, your mind focused, and your emotions are balanced, plateaus trigger full-body energy orgasms.

Channels

Targeting sweet spots feels good because it releases kundalini. The sexual energy moves around and massages the inside of your body. With practice you can direct it by *running energy*. And sometimes it blossoms on its own by *streaming* throughout your body.

Kundalini can also follow subtle energy channels in the body like those that connect the chakras.

You can intensify your excitement by connecting two sweet spots energetically, such as your jewels and a nipple, your G-spot and your lips, or your vajra (penis) and scrotum. We call these *hot links*, energy channels that you create inside your body.

Pleasure soars even more when you hook together a sweet spot in each of your bodies. That's why joining your jewels feels so good. We call energy channels that exchange kundalini between the two of you *passion circuits*.

Opening two passion circuits creates an *energy circle*. For example, energy flowing from his vajra into her yoni (vagina) streams up to her heart. She feels an outpouring of love that impacts his heart so he feels his heart energy and can create a circle to her heart. Which makes his vajra hotter and harder, and so on.

Phases

As we're getting started, we want to make sure you're tracking the five phases that Supernatural Sex cycles through:

- Phase 1: Loveplay
- Phase 2: Initial Entry
- Phase 3: The Valley
- Phase 4: Climbing
- Phase 5: Closing

As we mentioned, we prefer the more generic term *loveplay* for phase 1 to acknowledge that sometimes all you need is a hand, mouth, or toy to get satisfied. Loveplay is about connecting your souls first, then your hearts and minds, and finally your bodies. That results in erections for both men and women.

Initial entry, phase 2, is when a vajra first penetrates a yoni. You may say when a penis enters a vagina, but we prefer the more spiritual Tantric term jewel union. Though it doesn't last long, we deem it a unique phase because introducing something into such a sensitive orifice can be so intense. Initial entry also applies to anal sex. To avoid both medical and dirty words, we refer to that as *rosetta* sex. It looks a bit like a little rose, don't you think?

Supernatural lovers spend most of their time in phase 3, the Valley, stretching out their fun as long as they want. This phase got its name because arousal typically flattens out after the initial thrill. Instead of rushing toward orgasm, here you aim to fill your pleasure balloon, exchange more sexual electricity, and reach longer and stronger peaks.

When you decide to go for the Big O (orgasm), you shift into Climbing at phase 4 by going even higher. Though Supernatural Sex is orgasmic much of time, this is where you consciously decide to go for an explosive climax. You shift your focus here from the volume of pleasure flowing through your passion channels to increasing the electrical voltage, speed, and intensity of your sensations.

Phase 5, Closing, is a little ceremony in which you relax, wind down romantically, and set the stage for next time.

Orgasms

You probably think of orgasm as the climax of pleasure centered in the jewels and accompanied by a few seconds of pelvic contractions. Sex researchers in the last century defined it as the explosive release of tension due to the buildup of sexual excitement.

When you climax, your heart rate, breathing, and blood pressure spike. Your muscles, especially around your crotch, convulse rhythmically five to twelve times within ten to twenty seconds. You're probably wrapped up in waves of love and bliss from the outpouring of feel-good hormones. If you're the least bit uninhibited, you may well cry out, move, and shake.

This certainly describes the physical phenomena of orgasm. But we learned that there can be spiritual things going on, too. You might be engulfed in a sense of wonder. You may find yourself consumed with the rapture of union with your beloved. Or you may find yourself levitated into a state of oneness with the Divine.

Tantric *energy orgasms* include everything above but without the tension release. They're more than just tripping the right lever to blow off steam.

Energy orgasms are more spiritual, more an altered state of consciousness, a portal into a trance of non-ordinary reality like you can achieve through dreaming or meditation. They're an opening of your inner self, an outpouring of love, an energy connection at multiple levels of heart, mind, and soul.

Sure, it's wonderful when you're overtaken by an irresistible crescendo of passion. But since quick physical orgasm isn't the goal of Supernatural Sex, this book focuses more on the Valley phase rather than the Climbing phase.

Summary and Action Steps

These introductory comments are just setting the stage. To make sure you can put into action what's coming later, we suggest you stop for a moment and answer the following questions:

- Can you recall times when you felt kundalini alive and moving within you? How did it feel?
- What are your most sensitive sexual sweet spots?
- What causes your strongest sexual peaks and how do you handle them?
- When you're making love, how long do you typically spend in the Valley?
- What usually brings you to orgasmic peaks?

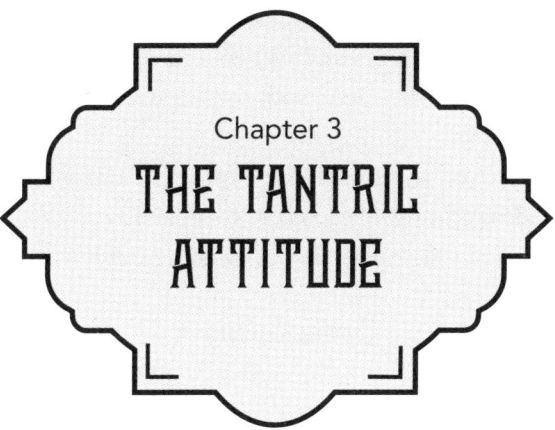

Chapter 3
THE TANTRIC ATTITUDE

Adopting the "Tantric attitude" helps build a solid platform for Supernatural Sex.[1]

The Tantric attitude is a decidedly sex-positive mindset but much more. You embrace the Tantric attitude when you say yes to pleasure, stay conscious, relax, feel your body, drop your goals, build intimacy, take responsibility for your own satisfaction, and treat everything about love and sex as sacred.

Saying Yes to Pleasure

The Tantric attitude is based on the premise that at your core you are a blissful spiritual being. Therefore, nothing is more important than feeling good.

Learn to celebrate your lusty, loving, childish, and mature desires as healthy. If this doesn't come easily, you may need to practice saying yes to pleasure instead of resisting it.

Allow things to happen, don't fight them. When you clearly hear your inner voice saying no to something, this includes heeding that guidance.

Let's say, for example, that your sweetie suggests trying rosetta (anal) sex. If you knee-jerk and freak out, you block any chance of building sexual energy. If you're not interested, by all means, say no. Only consenting to what you really want is fundamental in Supernatural Sex. But, if you're the least bit curious, you could negotiate a comfortable and safe way to experiment.

---

1. Margot Anand, *The Art of Sexual Ecstasy* (Los Angeles: Tarcher, 1989), 42–46.

A useful way to welcome pleasure instead of judging it is by using what Zen masters call the *beginner's mind*. When you operate with the beginner's mind, you approach new situations with openness, eagerness, and as few preconceptions as possible.

You'll know that you've adopted the Tantric attitude when your knee-jerk reaction to new ideas is to openly consider them and look forward to any possible pleasure instead of judging harshly or avoiding stubbornly.

Consciousness

The Tantric attitude is based on consciousness. The popular term for this today is *mindfulness*, which means being here now, awake inside, and aware of your surroundings.

Doesn't that sound completely different than thinking about baseball or what color you want to paint the bedroom when you're making love?

The energy practices of Supernatural Sex depend on you being fully conscious of what's happening both inside and out. So instead of just thinking, pay more attention. Instead of worrying, witness your actual responses. Instead of expecting your partner to react like they did last time, notice how they're behaving now.

The best way to raise consciousness is by practicing meditation. Meditation is a no-mind condition where you seek a deep sense of inner peace filled with stillness. But trying to empty your head of chattering thoughts is quite challenging.

We're as human as most people. Jeffre is easily distracted if the temperature or music isn't just right. Somraj's mind tends to wander to how hard his erection is and how close he is to coming.

Fortunately, gurus have developed meditation techniques down the ages that can help you quiet your mind and be more present while making love. Here's our basic practice.

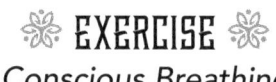
Conscious Breathing

1. Sit comfortably and focus on your breath.
2. Feel the air coming in through your nose, moving down into your lungs, rising up, and then being expelled.

3. When extraneous thoughts pop up, simply shift your attention back to what your breath is doing and how it feels.

Relaxation

It's natural to tense up when you get sexually excited. Unfortunately, that prevents sexual energy from flowing smoothly. Remember, kundalini moves in subtle channels. That's why relaxation, especially when you're highly aroused, is a critical foundation of Supernatural Sex.

Being relaxed means to chill out, stay comfortable, and calm yourself. Stressed, uptight, and on edge is the opposite.

When you relax, your blood circulates freely, your nerve circuits open wide, and your mind slows. That's the only way you can feel sensations, melt into pleasure, savor your turn-on, and float away on clouds of ecstasy.

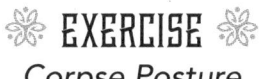
EXERCISE
Corpse Posture

1. A great way to start practicing relaxation is with the yoga corpse posture. To do this, just lie down, relax all your muscles, and don't move.
2. Anytime you find yourself tensing up, consciously tighten and relax each muscle or part of the body.
3. It helps if you imagine your in-breaths bathing each muscle and your out-breaths releasing any tension.

We're not against the common practice of having a couple of alcoholic drinks or tokes of cannabis to get relaxed before sex. But too much can lessen your awareness, sensitivity, and conscious energy control at first. We suggest you learn to relax cold turkey before experimenting with stimulants.

Feel Your Body

Consciousness and relaxation put you in a place where you can feel your body. Without that, you'll never be able to master your kundalini.

New Age folks call this *being in your body*. To fully be in your body, center yourself in your heart, open your senses, feel more, and think less.

Practicing *sensate focus* helps. That means tuning in to all your senses: taste, touch, sight, sound, and smell. The more you train yourself to focus on your sensations, the more sensitive you'll become.

Have you ever felt lighter or heavier while making love? Have you ever had goose bumps or heat flush flood your skin? Have you ever felt shudders spreading from your groin down your legs or up your torso? Noticing these things is sensate focus.

Getting better at being in your body starts with accepting it, even loving it. Take your clothes off and look in a full-length mirror. How does it make you feel? What thoughts run through your mind?

An essential premise of the Tantric attitude is that your body is a divine gift. Don't buy into the media's unrealistic standards of beauty. Learn to honor your body and your beloved's. Treat your body well. Celebrate it as a holy temple.

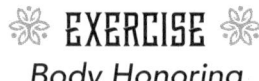

EXERCISE
Body Honoring

1. To practice together, undress each other and, one at a time, touch your partner all over.
2. Receivers, report the thoughts and sensations you have from each stroke. Find some positive thoughts about each body part and speak them out loud.
3. Givers, add your own compliments and appreciations.
4. Eventually you'll want to practice sensate focus in the throes of lovemaking. Occasionally slow down and savor the sensations in your body. You might briefly mention what you're feeling and where those sensations are.

Drop Goals and Surrender

Supernatural Sex is about feeling as much pleasure as possible for as long as you can. It's not about climaxing as fast as you can.

If you have sex with a goal, such as making yourself or your sweetie have a Big O, it takes you out of the moment where all the sensations lie. It puts you in your head, not in your body. It creates pressure instead of letting you relax into pleasure.

To drop your goals, enter into lovemaking without a target, plan, time frame, or agenda. Focus on welcoming whatever happens with as few expectations as possible. Enjoy what you're feeling instead of measuring how well things are going and figuring out what to do next.

Learn to *surrender* to whatever happens. That doesn't mean give up. It means letting things be instead of trying to control the outcome. Somraj learned to drop his goals and surrender during jewel union (sexual intercourse) using the following exercise.

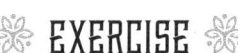

EXERCISE
Last Stroke Technique

1. The next time you make love, remind yourself to savor the sensations that each stroke creates as if they were the last time you'd ever feel them.
2. When his vajra is sliding into her yoni or rosetta, put all your attention on how it feels in that exact moment. As his vajra slides out, simply appreciate how wonderful it is.
3. Don't think about what's next. Then, when there is another stroke, be grateful and cherish the next surge of excitement.

If you knew that this thrust was going to be the last ever, wouldn't you want to make it last? Wouldn't you want to feel it to the hilt (pun intended)? Wouldn't you take it slow and savor the sensations of each and every millimeter?

The Last Stroke Technique is also useful when things are getting too intense, if you need to catch your breath, or just to spread out the energy so it's not confined in your jewels.

Intimacy

Intimacy is when you feel close, comfortable, and bonded at multiple levels. It's when you feel warmth, affinity, and a sense of togetherness with another person. It's when you feel safe enough to be yourself because you know that you won't be judged, criticized, or put down. It's when you reveal who you really are and how you really feel.

Intimacy is a true heart connection.

You're truly intimate when you trust enough to let your partner see inside. You'll only do this when you know you'll be loved and accepted whatever you say and do.

Are you motivated to be spiritually naked in front of each other? That means dropping pretensions, coming clean, and showing up for real.

Deep intimacy is an essential component of the Tantric attitude. The more you talk, open up, and reveal, the more intimacy you'll create.

Heart meditation is an easy way to improve your intimacy. The Heart Meditation Exercise is similar to the breath-following Conscious Breathing Exercise we suggested earlier. But this one focuses on your heart connection instead of your breath alone.

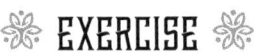

EXERCISE
Heart Meditation

1. Sit across from each other and make eye contact.
2. Breathe in unison and feel the love that binds you.
3. Continue eye-gazing and breathing this way for a few minutes to deepen your intimate connection.

Though it's a sweet thing to do, you don't have to physically press your chests against each other. It's a matter of focusing on your heart connection with the person in front of you. It's more about intention and awareness than action.

When you're heart-connected, you'll feel emotional rapport, mental accord, and an overall sense of harmony. Try this while you're making love and you'll understand the meaning of the term *heart-centered*.

Personal Responsibility

Sometimes it's great to be taken. Your lover wants you so badly that you revel in surrendering to their love and desire. This can be especially powerful if you're engrossed in a romantic fantasy.

Supernatural Sex doesn't always operate that way. A key element of that difference is that you both take full responsibility for your own pleasure.

You need to act as the foremost expert of your own turn-ons. That means you know your body, what it wants in each moment, and ask for it. You offer enthusiastic consent when you choose and withhold it when you're not getting what you want.

Responsibility means monitoring your own comfort, adjusting your position if needed, and asking for changes. You don't hesitate to shift where your playmate's leg, elbow, hand, mouth, vajra, or toy is hitting you. You gracefully communicate your desires and diplomatically steer each other toward what feels best.

One vital foundation of the Tantric attitude is personal responsibility. When you take charge of your own pleasure, your sharing will be more real. And when you trust in yourself, you can devote yourself to giving pleasure at the same time.

Personal responsibility in the bedroom requires that you both ask for what you want whenever you need to. Unless you become an expert in your own pleasure, how can you be assured that you will get it?

Supernatural lovers study what brings them the most pleasure. What do each of your erogenous zones desire in different situations? What triggers which kinds of orgasm? What is uncomfortable and painful? Answering these questions requires experimenting with your own body using the beginner's mind.

We're advocating Tantric masturbation, which is about increasing and extending pleasure. We call it *self-pleasuring* to distinguish it from simply getting yourself off as fast as possible.

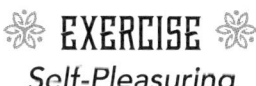

EXERCISE
Self-Pleasuring

1. To practice pleasuring yourself, start with a gentle touch all over.
2. Explore places that don't get much attention during sex. As you discover areas that give you good feelings, linger and savor the sensations.
3. When your jewels ask for it, gradually shift your attention to erotic massage. Play around to find out what feels best and enjoy it for as long as you want. Use lubrication to avoid chafing and to enhance your sensations.
4. After a while, add some sex toys if you want.

5. Take your time and enjoy. If your body asks for release or any kind of climax, go for it.

Self-pleasuring is a great way to experiment with new turn-ons like softer or harder touch and slower or faster strokes. You can play with awakening new responses from ignored nipples, scrotum, yoni lips, or rosettas. Be sure to note anything new, notable, or valuable and pass it on to your beloved.

From practicing over the years, we have increased our sensitivity to many sensations. Somraj once thought he didn't have any sensation in his nipples, but after regular attention they're awakening.

Even better, do this exercise in front of each other. With the Tantric attitude, that can be really hot and open your physical and energy bodies to the eruption of kundalini.

Sacred Sex as a Gift

There's one more question you need to answer to fully embrace the Tantric attitude. In your mind do you view sex as dirty and sinful or as a sacred, spiritual act?

In Tantra, we don't separate the physical from the sacred. Here are Jeffre's views on sacred sex with special emphasis for women.

Recently, one of my favorite romance authors announced that, in response to reader requests, she would be offering "clean" versions of her novels. In other words, the hot sex scenes that I loved so much would be watered down and occur behind closed doors. Then the reader wouldn't be confronted with the rawness of real sex.

My heart sank when I read this because I knew I'd no longer read her once-juicy novels. But even more important was the reality that prompted this change. In spite of being addicted to romance, many women don't enjoy sex. As a result, they don't want to be reminded of women who do.

Too few people believe that sex is good and healthy for spiritual, physical, and psychological reasons. Some people believe if they were more spiritual they would be nonsexual. Our Tantric attitude is quite the reverse.

Can you feel the sacredness of sex? Or is there a hidden voice in your head that argues with that view?

I am blessed to be human. I revere whatever divine force created and animated me. All parts of my existence are sacred. That includes my body.

When I'm sexual, it feels spiritual, too. And when I'm spiritual, it feels sexual. It's all sacred.

Sadly, far too many people still feel guilty, shame themselves, and condemn sex except for procreation. If you embrace your human faculties, such as your brain, heart, digestion, and reproductive systems, as being miracles, can't you include sexuality in that list?

Since you are a spiritual being, you can learn to honor your sexual parts, desires, and ability to give and receive pleasure. To become more sex positive, take an honest inventory of your beliefs about pleasure. Think back to where they originally came from and compare them to how you feel now. Often counseling or energy healing can help you release programming that is blocking your pleasure.

Can you thank the universe, the source, or the god you worship that you have the capacity to feel the amazing joys of physical intimacy with a beloved? And each time you have an orgasm? It's a sacred miracle when you dive in deep and feel the love of the universe coursing through your sexual self this way.

I want to shout my thanks from the rooftops. Will you join me?

Elevate your wants to the sacred level. Please allow yourself the permission to express your ecstatic self. Then allow yourself to revel in the beauty of this miraculous physical, mental, and spiritual life we are given.

It's all good! Because it's all divine, sacred, and spiritual.

Summary and Action Steps

- Practice saying yes to pleasure instead of resisting it.
- Meditate using the Conscious Breathing Exercise.
- Learn to relax with the Corpse Posture.
- Improve your sensate focus.
- Celebrate your physical form with the Body Honoring Exercise.
- Drop your goals and enter into sex with as few expectations as possible so you can create your experience as you go.
- Practice the Last Stroke Technique while touching or making love.

- Build more intimacy with the Heart Meditation.
- Take responsibility for your own pleasure by practicing self-pleasuring regularly.
- Release your negative beliefs about sex and hold it in your heart, mind, and soul as sacred.

Chapter 4
PARTNERING

Supernatural Sex requires a cooperative style of loving that we call *partnering*. That's different than the kind of ordinary sex where one partner, typically the man, acts like he knows it all and takes total charge. Such one-sided power only happens if his playmate passively lets him have his way.

Playing out domination and submission fantasies can be fun. But will he truly know what she needs to be fulfilled? Will he be able to lose himself in orgasmic rapture at the same time?

Further, making love as isolated islands insulated from each other creates minimal energy connection.

Supernatural Sex is a consensual act where you play together. It's equal cooperation, not a performance that one does to the other. One of you isn't active all the time while the other is passive. You share leadership. Two empowered partners are necessary.

The partnership starts when you both look honestly at your inner desires. Until you each hear and communicate an enthusiastic yes to connect, you should go no further. Cooperation like this depends on taking responsibility, speaking up, and paying attention to your own sensations.

It's freeing when you trust each other to speak up. Then you don't have to worry if you're pleasing or hurting each other. If his vajra is jabbing a tender spot, he wants to know immediately. If he's getting too close to the edge, she wants to know now.

When you trust each other to look after yourself and communicate, it's easier to relax, get fully into your body, and sink into pleasure.

Of course, caring partners also tune in to the one they're with. Though you're ultimately responsible for your own pleasure, you're also there to support your beloved. Listening, watching, and sensing what's going on over there allows you to help your playmate's quest for ecstasy.

Tuning In to Your Stereo

Loving partners make love in stereo. One channel is tuned to yourself while the other is tuned to your playmate. If you're used to focusing on just one of you, or if your mind wanders incessantly, this double focus can be a challenge.

That's why something like the 69 position with simultaneous oral sex is easier said than done. You have to divide your attention between what you're doing and what you're feeling. That's one of the reasons we love jewel union when we're both sending and receiving kundalini at the same time. What's pleasing one of us automatically pleases the other.

Certainly, there are monaural moments like when we first get turned-on. Then we focus more on the single channel of the pleasure we're receiving. But when our excitement grows, we naturally reach out for our partner's energy. Uniting the giving and receiving channels is a gift of Supernatural Sex. When we make love in stereo, we sense that what's pleasing one of us is simultaneously pleasing the other.

We exchange roles frequently. Jeffre might take the initiative by giving Somraj oral sex. Then he throws her on her back and plunges inside. She pushes him over and mounts him. He rolls her over and licks her yoni until she demands that his vajra enters her again. We spiral back and forth from top to bottom, dominant and submissive, leading and following.

Even when Somraj is on top in the classic missionary position, this partnership is alive. Because he's paying attention, he's receptive to her pleasure flows. His sexual stroking follows her hip rhythms, her moans, and her muscle contractions.

When she wants it slower, he follows. When she wants it deeper or faster, he senses it and complies. Or she gently asks, "deeper please" or forcefully demands, "fuck me hard now!"

In Supernatural Sex you both generate kundalini, guide each other to fill your pleasure balloons, and exchange sexual energy. This requires that some of your attention is always on yourself and some is always on your playmate.

About the Partnering Questions

An easy way to each take responsibility for your partnership is by discussing three *partnering questions* before the action heats up. These questions address the following:

1. desires
2. concerns
3. boundaries

Communicating about these three issues is vital to create a relationship of mutual consent, energy balance, full participation, and equal giving and receiving.

First, share your *desires* by explaining what you want, intend, or hope will happen. Do you want a quickie or a longie? Multiple orgasms would be great if your energy holds up. Is this true love or just a one-night stand?

Next, raise any *concerns* or worries on your mind. This could include safer sex, sex history, birth control, privacy, confidentially, or health issues. "Should I wear a condom?" "My lower back is sore." "Let's use a towel because my period is coming on."

Finally, set any *boundaries* that are needed. What lines don't you want to cross and what specific acts don't you want to engage in right now? "We can't wake up the kids." "Anal isn't an option tonight." "Sorry, but I never do oral."

When you each answer the partnering questions and discuss whatever comes up, you'll feel safer and freer to play full out. If it bothers you how premeditated this seems, remember that Supernatural Sex is willful. Your minds and souls are leading, not your hormones.

In the real world, the issues raised by the partnering questions are a moving target. Keep this dialogue going as needed. When you keep the decks clear, your minds can stay focused on the fun and your hearts can remain open without any hidden anxieties or expectations.

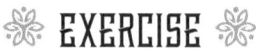

EXERCISE
Partnering Questions Discussion

1. Discuss the partnering questions the next time you make love. First, think about what you want to do, feel, or give, as well as any issues that come up.
2. Next, share your desires, concerns, and boundaries. The listener should simply pay attention, acknowledge what was said, and only chime in with questions or clarifications.
3. One of you can answer all three questions at once, or you can alternate discussing each question before moving on to the next.

Verbal and Nonverbal Communication

Sex like that of hungry wild animals can be an exciting way to start a relationship, but lust isn't a solid enough foundation for a long-term partnership. You need authentic nonverbal and verbal communication to take full responsibility for your side of the partnership. It strengthens your intimacy when you need it most. When you show your passion, your breath, sounds, and body motions speak loudly and count as part of this communication.

Isn't it great when your lover is bucking and moaning and showing you what's really turning them on without words? When Jeffre pushes back, Somraj knows she wants it harder and deeper and complies. When Somraj suddenly starts shaking, Jeffre knows he's enjoying an energy orgasm and hangs on.

Communicating via body language is best because it keeps you out of your head. But it isn't always enough. Sometimes you have to ask for what you want. Sometimes you have to give feedback, coach, or redirect your sweetie's fingers, mouth, body, or jewels.

Supernatural Sex relies on an energy connection as well as a physical one. When you're holding back things you need to say, you may close down those subtle channels. When you're withholding vital information for fear of hurting your partner's feelings, they won't know how to plug into your kundalini.

We know that sexual communication is difficult. Even when things are going well, it's a challenge to talk about intimate things like private parts, pleasure, and orgasms. But it is essential and gets easier the more you do it.

In spite of the romance novel fantasy that your dream lover always knows the perfect thing to do, reality is different. Sometimes we need guidance. For example, Jeffre once had a lover who couldn't seem to get the knack of the kind of oral sex she preferred. At a neutral time away from bed, she explained what she wanted. He agreed to let her guide his mouth until he got it. They were both thrilled at the pleasure he learned to give her.

Communication Tools

The partnering questions start communication on the right foot. But you need to keep it going. Here are a few more tools that can keep you in sync.

Use *sweet everythings* to lavish compliments and appreciation on each other. Doesn't that sound better than sweet nothings? The simplest is when you moan, "Yes, yes, yes" or "Oh, wow!" Also try "I love you" or "That feels so good," or "You're so strong," or "You're so beautiful when you come," or "I love it when you fuck me like that."

But what if your arousal level changes, you want something different, or you're struck by an irresistible kinky whim? Constructive *feedback* and sincere requests sandwiched between sweet everythings help keep your playtime on track.

To give feedback you might say, "Oooh, that's way hot! Do that some more," or "My lower leg is getting numb. Can you shift your weight? Great, that's much better," or "I feel like I need something different, like some long, deep, slow strokes for a bit. *(moans)* Way yummy!"

Another way to keep communication flowing is by *checking in*. If one of you is wondering what's going on, ask a *yes-no question* like "Faster?" or "Too much?" or "More?"

A good time to check in is right before any major change in speed, position, or direction. You could ask, "Want to spread your legs so I can get on top?" Or before entering your honey's yoni or rosetta with fingers or vajra, you could check, "Is your yoni/rosetta ready for a visit?" Or "I'm getting really close to coming. Okay if I slow down for a bit?"

Sometimes you need more guidance than a shake of the head can convey. Then try an *open-ended question* like, "Which position would be best for your sore back?" or "What would your yoni/vajra/rosetta like now?" or "Your energy seems a little low. What can I do to help?"

Check-ins are helpful when one of you is unclear or needs some information. If you see an unexpected expression on your playmate's face, ask, "What's up?" If your lover's sounds, breathing, or motions suddenly change, you might check in with, "What just happened?" Or if his erection is waning, she might ask, "What would your vajra like now?"

These questions prompt you to look inside and keep your partner informed about what's going on. Used appropriately, they strengthen your presence, increase your confidence, and keep you in sync.

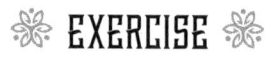
Communication Tools

1. The next time you make love, include the above communication tools in your discussion of the partnering questions (desires, concerns, boundaries).
2. Talk about how you might use sweet everythings, constructive feedback, sincere requests, check-ins, and open-ended questions to better synchronize what you do together.
3. Afterward discuss how the tools worked and what might be better.

Creating a Sacred Space

The platform for Supernatural Sex isn't ready until you fashion a *sacred space* together. That means consecrating the place you make love into a hallowed ground by taking conscious care with love and divine connection. Physically, that includes cleaning and decorating. Emotionally, that includes being present, expressing affection, and communicating openly.[2]

Sometimes our sacred space is the bedroom and sometimes it's a futon in front of the fireplace. On special occasions we rent a luxurious hotel room and dress it up. You can set up a sacred space anywhere free of distractions where you're both comfortable and feel free to be uninhibited. If you've got kids or parents or roommates behind a thin wall, this may take some creativity.

Before the action heats up, we like to exchange *namastés*, the traditional Indian greeting where we bring our palms together over our chests and bow. Sometimes we connect with a *heart bonding* where we lock our eyes together

---

2. Margot Anand, *The Art of Sexual Ecstasy* (Los Angeles: Tarcher, 1989), 68.

with a hand over each other's chest. Often, we do a shamanic ritual by acknowledging the four directions and calling in the energies we want in our space.

The few moments creating a sacred space together puts your attention on your heart and soul connection. It demonstrates how important you are to each other, so your engagement will be sweet, sacred, and hot from the get-go.

❦ EXERCISE ❦
Sacred Space

1. The next time you make love, start by creating a sacred space together that appeals to all your senses and activates the energy from all your chakras.
2. Make sure it's warm enough.
3. Collect oils, lubes, and toys so you won't be interrupted later.
4. Bring finger foods, wine, and fresh water.
5. Light candles, burn incense, and play some sensual music.
6. Afterward discuss how creating a sacred space impacted your lovemaking.

Summary and Action Steps

- Play together as partners.
- Look inside at your desires, ask for what you want, and pay attention to your playmate.
- Make love in stereo, alternating between leading and following.
- Discuss the partner questions before you engage in Supernatural Sex.
- The more you open your sexual communication to deepen your intimacy, the easier it gets.
- Lavish sweet everythings on your partner.
- Give feedback when you get out of sync or want something different.
- Check in with yes-no or open-ended questions.
- Create a sacred space together before you make love.

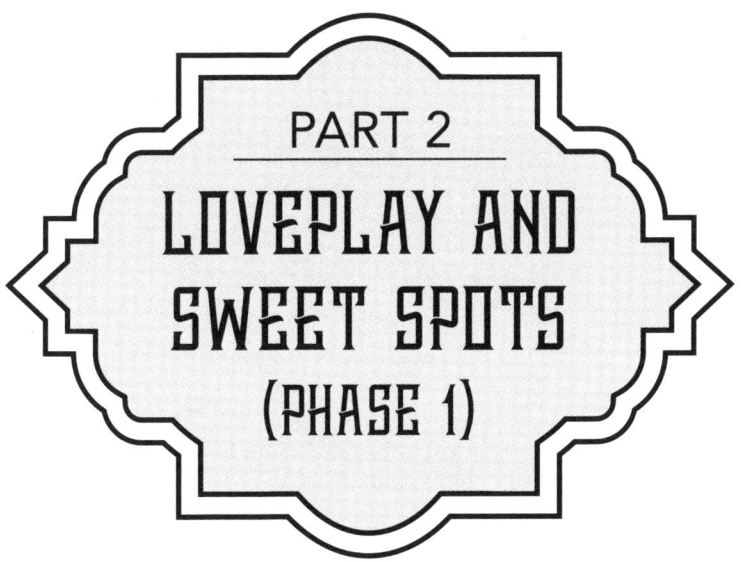

PART 2
LOVEPLAY AND SWEET SPOTS
(PHASE 1)

To excel at Supernatural Sex, you need to develop a healthy relationship with your own and your lover's private parts.

Your jewels, whether vajra (penis), yoni (vulva and vagina), or rosetta (anus), possess a natural magnetism. They contain positive and negative poles that emit strong attractive bioelectric energies.

Some say that the magnetism is animal while others claim it's a divine sacrament. Or is it sexual chemistry? Whatever it is activates your mind, hormones, and spirit to draw you together and turn you on. And sometimes not.

Erogenous zones are places that erupt with sensation when contacted. We call them *sweet spots*. The primary ones are around and inside a woman's yoni, a man's vajra, and the rosetta. Stimulating a sweet spot causes kundalini to stream out and shower the body with pleasure.

In the next three chapters we're going to explore sexual arousal and the fifty physical sweet spots associated with the sexual organs (twenty for men and thirty for women).

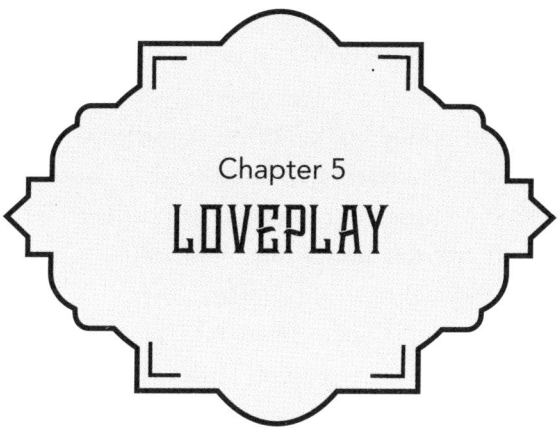

Chapter 5
LOVEPLAY

Have you ever seen the bumper sticker "Put your mind in gear before your mouth is engaged"? In Supernatural Sex, that changes to "Arouse your mind and spirit before you engage your jewels."

Arousal is getting turned-on enough to make your body excited. It's when your sexual juices start flowing, including liquid, chemical, electrical, and magnetic. It's when your skin craves contact, especially your jewels. It's when your senses get awakened and heighten your sensitivity and your mind gets consumed with sexual pleasure. It's when your brain, nerves, and metabolism reach out for more and more stimuli.

Before engaging in jewel union, it's fundamental that you both get thoroughly aroused first. That's the purpose of this chapter.

Getting Turned-On

Getting turned-on is a multilevel experience. You need to be spiritually ready. You have to feel safe. Your heart must be willing to open. Your body has to say yes. You have to shift your mind into the right gear. And then you need to announce your enthusiastic consent before anything happens.

When all of that's a go, you enter into each other's personal space. Your biofields engage even before your bodies do. Then, when your lips, fingers, skin, and jewels touch, energy starts flowing. Heat, electricity, hunger, sweat, and other juices erupt.

As you reach a peak of pleasure, your heart flutters, your eyes glaze over, your metabolism speeds up, and your brain triggers the release of hormones.

Uninhibited lovers also experience curling toes, wriggling hips, arching backs, shivers down the spine, exaggerated facial expressions, sensual moans, expressive groans, and uninhibited gasps.

Arousal affects your entire body. The more turned-on you get, the more sensitive you become to touch and the less sensitive to pain. Your breathing accelerates, your blood pressure spikes, your heart rate increases, and your muscles get tense. You'll probably notice this more around your arms, legs, face, and pelvic region as they collect erotic charge.

Vasocongestion occurs in an organ when more blood is flowing in than out. When you get turned-on, vasocongestion causes your skin, especially around your chest, neck, face, hands, and feet, to get warmer, darker, and redder. This *sex flush*, which is more common with women than men, also increases perspiration. It's vasocongestion, blood flooding your jewels, that causes erections. The nipples of most women, and some men, also get erect.

Arousal is limited if you're not feeling good or aren't in the right mood. Your libido has to be alive and well to feel desire. This sex drive in both genders is regulated and fueled by the hormone testosterone. As you age, both sexes go through some form of menopause that causes the production of this essential natural substance to drop off. Not to fear though. Our physician has prescribed supplements that allow us to give and receive as much sexual pleasure as when we were young.

The above is more the medical story about arousal than the energetic one. The Tantric view is that the pooling and flowing of kundalini is what accounts for sexual turn-on.

Loveplay

Loveplay is any kind of intimate, physical interaction that demonstrates desire and stimulates turn-on.

Loveplay in Supernatural Sex starts with the upper chakras, opening your hearts to love, meditating together, connecting at a soul level, and getting your minds in their proper low-key but focused gear. That's the purpose of the Tantric attitude, especially the partnering questions and creating a sacred space.

Or maybe sexting is your thing.

Physical arousal begins with the many delicious ways to titillate your lover's body. The skin is the biggest erogenous zone. The average human body is encased in thirty-five hundred square inches of skin. That's a lot of inches to play with.

Sensual massage everywhere, even when it bypasses the jewels, gradually gets our motors running by fully awakening our senses. Because we've learned to relax, receive, and open to the natural flow of sexual energy, we only need a few minutes of erotic touch to get Jeffre wet and Somraj hard.

The *Kama Sutra* suggested lots of ways to titillate lots of places around the body. Another Indian love manual, the sixteenth-century *Ananga Ranga*, taught that a woman's erogenous zones include the crown of the head, scalp, hair, center of forehead, eyelids, eyebrows, temples, cheeks, mouth, lips, ears, neck, throat, shoulders, chest, breasts, nipples, belly, navel, waist, fingers, hands, arms, armpits, sides, back, butt, thighs, legs, knees, feet, ankles, and toes.

We call these thirty-three spots secondary sweet spots.

In our trainings we've noticed that many men touch women harder and faster than women like. To combat this, we teach *Tantric touch*: light, slow, tender skin-to-skin contact with full consciousness. It's very differernt than deep therapeutic massage. Giving and receiving Tantric touch is how you can train your nervous systems to become galvanized with sexual electricity through the slightest, subtlest touch.

As the following exercise demonstrates, sensual massage with Tantric touch is an exercise in applying the Tantric attitude.

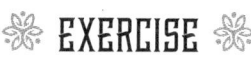

EXERCISE
Tantric Touch

1. Giver, make it a point to be totally present, totally conscious, and totally attentive to what you're doing.
2. Feel every contact fully, visualizing energy flowing as warm golden light through your fingers and sparking across your honey's skin.
3. Receiving Tantric touch is far from passive. As a receiver, enter a calm, relaxed state and reach out with your senses. Be totally present to the feelings and sensations you experience.
4. Visualize the energy flow coming into your body.

The more you practice Tantric touch, the more sensitive you'll become to each other's energy.

Other Turn-Ons

One of Jeffre's favorite forms of loveplay is deep, wet kissing. Kissing is so wonderful because it stimulates so many chakras. Your vision, minds, and third eyes are totally focused on each other. You're exchanging breath. You can feel each other's heart beating. You're immersed in each other's personal space.

Kissing all parts of the body is also delicious. Alternating mouth and hand caresses can be a great combo. You might find the strongest responses from kissing the head, face, neck, sides, back, butt, hands, feet, and inner thighs. Women especially love their breasts massaged and their nipples squeezed, pulled, and twirled. Sometimes we get a good jolt from tapping, kissing, blowing, or humming on our chakras.

Even though the skin is the biggest erogenous zone, the mind is the strongest. We've seen impressive displays of auto-eroticism where people turn themselves on without any physical contact. Like us, do you get a charge out of erotica, fantasies, or porn?

Devotees of the *Kama Sutra* specialized in sensuous scratching, biting, and slapping. If your desires run hotter, bondage, domination, and role-playing might be your route to super turn-on.

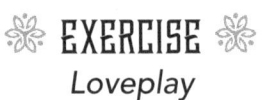

EXERCISE
Loveplay

1. Talk about what kinds of loveplay most turn you on.
2. Demonstrate what you like on your own body.
3. Experiment on each other using fingers first and then maybe sex toys. Cover your honey's entire body, checking in with each other as you progress.
4. When your playmate is turned-on enough, begin caressing, nuzzling, flicking, stroking, fingering, grabbing, pulling, licking, and sucking the jewels.
5. Don't be in a hurry. Major in savoring every sensation and see how long you can make them last.

Don't follow the same agenda every time. Variety, spontaneity, and playfulness are your best loveplay guides.

Erections

Sexual arousal produces tense, hot, and swollen erections in both men and women. An *erection* occurs when the brain sends signals to your jewels, causing them to fill with blood or become *engorged*. That's why they swell and darken. When they get tense, hot, and swollen, you could also say they are *tumescent*.

Whenever tissues get engorged or tumescent, sensitivity to touch soars.

When a man's vajra gets rigid, sticks out, and stands up, it's easy to tell that he has an erection. You may not notice that his testicles might also increase in size by 50 percent or more.

Women get erections, too. There is a complex network of parts buried inside a woman's groin that get engorged from sexual stimulation. Though it's not as obvious at first glance, when a woman's yoni becomes erect, it gets puffier and redder.

Both genders' rosettas can also grow erect. The sensitive anal tissues become congested with blood making them darken in color. Both yonis and rosettas may become moister from secretions and perspiration. The muscles surrounding the jewels begin twitching and contracting as well.

Lubrication

Many women secrete copious amounts of natural lubrication from the Bartholin's glands near the bottom of each side of the yoni. (See figure 6 on page 61.) Others don't emit much regardless of what you do. Lots of factors, including age, emotions, health, medications, and menopause influence how wet a woman gets when turned-on.

No doubt, slippery friction during loveplay and jewel union feels so much better than dry chafing. But being dry doesn't mean lack of excitement. Don't make a big deal about it. Fortunately, sex product manufacturers have invented substitute personal lubricants to bolster natural wetness. There are really two ways to go: oil and water.

Because oil-based lubes don't dry out quickly, we often use massage cream or thicker products for loveplay on a vajra or outer yoni. Some are petroleum-based like Vaseline, and some are silicone-based. The use of organic coconut oil is growing. Somraj's favorite for external self-pleasuring is a makeup remover found at many drugstores called Albolene.

There are two main drawbacks to oil-based lubes. First, they deteriorate latex by opening small pores that can allow the passage of viruses and bacteria. When you use a condom for protection against STDs (sexually transmitted diseases) or for birth control, don't use these thicker lubricants.

Second, we only use oil-based lubes on the outside. In other words, keep it away from yoni's mouth. The environment of inner yoni is a carefully balanced one, easily disturbed by unnatural substances. Any woman who's ever suffered from vaginal thrush will vehemently agree. Be careful not to introduce anything artificial or edible inside a yoni.

That includes digestibles like Vaseline, oil, fruit jelly, whipped cream, chocolate sauce, honey, or many feminine hygiene and spermicide products. One physician friend is so zealous about this that he urges women to never put anything inside their yoni that isn't pure water or skin.

Water-Based Lubes

Fortunately, the other major category of sexual lubricant, the water-based type, is great inside. Though it's not as thick nor as long-lasting as many commercial products, saliva is the most natural, plentiful, and inexpensive. And it's fun to apply.

Water-based lubes are more comfortable and better merge with a woman's inherent secretions. Some are thinner, some are thicker, and some are more readily absorbed. Unfortunately, they tend to dry out more quickly, which requires more frequent application or recharging with water spray.

There are lots of nonsaliva choices on the market today. Wet, Astroglide, Liquid Silk, and K-Y are some of the more commonly used ones. Our favorite is the thick version of Probe. It has a natural grapefruit-based preservative and is largely tasteless, which makes it great for oral sex, too.

The most outstanding advantage of Probe is that it has the same *osmolality* as skin. That means it doesn't suck moisture out of your tissues or force any of its ingredients through your pores.

Some lubes feel better and others are irritating. Make sure the lube you use pleases you both. That includes taste if you're inclined to switch to oral sex anytime. We encourage you to experiment with different products when you need to bolster your natural slipperiness.

❀ · ❀ · ❀

We've just touched the surface on all the fun things you can do for loveplay. Play around with words and actions that get you both in the mood (if you're not already). Many women need to get in the right emotional space before getting aroused. So be sure to start with intimacy before concentrating on stimulating the jewels as the next two chapters explain.

Summary and Action Steps

- Get each other fully aroused first.
- Use a wide variety of loveplay all over the body before jewel union.
- Use Tantric touch for heartfelt, sensitive, sensual massage.
- Experiment with different personal lubricants until you find what pleases you.

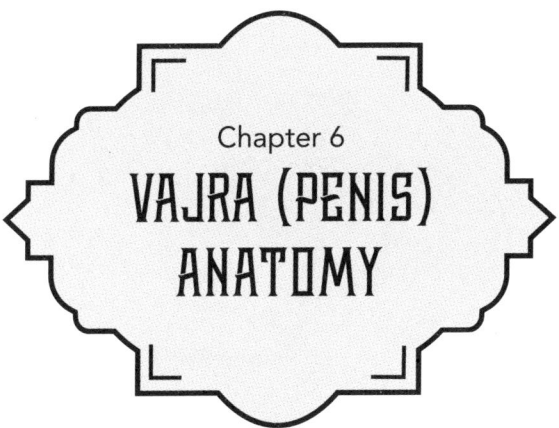

Chapter 6
VAJRA (PENIS) ANATOMY

To help you find and stimulate sweet spots, the next two chapters cover male and female sexual anatomy. This chapter will give you a firm grasp of the male penis. We prefer to use the Tibetan term *vajra*, which means *diamond thunderbolt* or *scepter of power*. Diamond for its hardness and thunderbolt for its divine qualities of injecting explosive kundalini.[3]

Vajras come in many shapes, colors, and sizes. Some are long and skinny, some are short and thick. As an introduction to choosing sexual positions, the *Kama Sutra* classified vajras according to their size. A *hare* was about five inches long, a *bull* was about seven, and a *horse* about ten. Surveys have shown that six inches is average in the modern world.

Unaltered vajras have *foreskin* that covers the head until erect or pulled back. Circumcised ones have had the foreskin removed surgically. All types and sizes of vajras work just fine. Size isn't everything. Fit, or relative size, is more important when considering penetration, as is the muscle tone of the yoni.

Vajra's Sweet Spots

Here is a short course in vajra anatomy: In spite of the common nickname *boner*, the male sex organ has no bones. Nor any muscles inside, either.

There are twenty sweet spots on and around a vajra. Though yours or your honey's might be sensitive everywhere, there are ten erogenous zones on the male organ itself and ten more in the vicinity.

Figure 3 on page 54 shows the twenty sweet spots on the male jewels.

---

3. Margot Anand, *The Art of Sexual Ecstasy* (Los Angeles: Tarcher, 1989), 215.

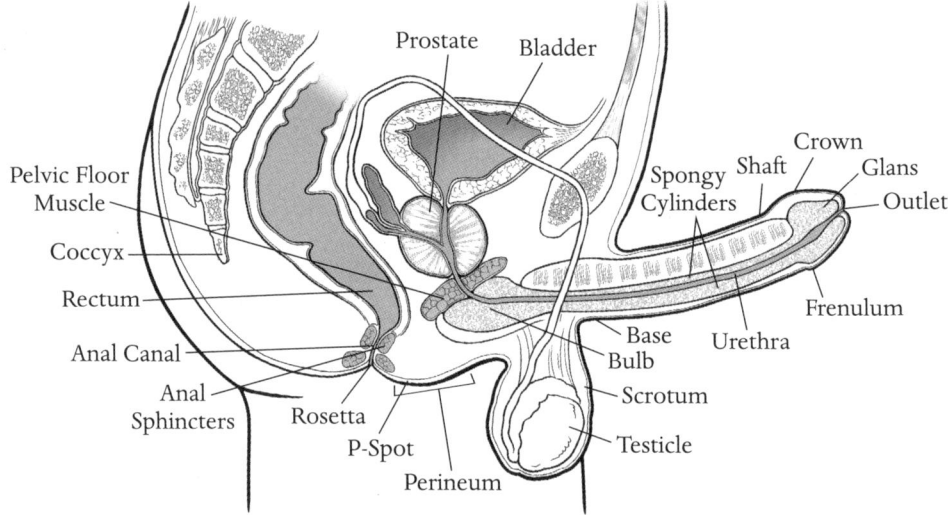

Figure 3: Male Jewels with Twenty Sweet Spots

1. The *shaft* is the long rod, noticeably longer and firmer when erect.
2. The *glans* is the smooth skin on vajra's head. It's highly sensitive due to its many nerve endings, almost as many as your fingertips.
3. We call the opening in the glans the *outlet* since that's how fluids exit the body. The medical name is *meatus*.
4. The *crown*, or *corona*, is the sensitive ridge that circles the bottom of the glans.
5. The *frenulum* is the highly sensitive soft tissue below the crown that connects the underside of the shaft to the glans.
6. Vajra's *base* is the lower part of the shaft closest to the body.
7. Figure 3 shows a circumcised male so the *foreskin*, the retractable fold of skin that covers vajra's head, doesn't appear.

Figure 3 also shows what's inside a vajra:

8. The *urethra* is the slender tube that transmits urine and semen out of the body. It extends from the bladder to the outlet at the tip of vajra's head.
9. The urethra is surrounded by three long *spongy cylinders* of erectile tissue that account for a vajra's ability to swell, harden, and lengthen when tumescent. Stimulating the urethra and its outlet can be pleasurable. But doing this internally can damage your tissues if not done carefully.
10. Vajra's *bulb* is the lowest part of vajra's shaft below the base and inside the body. You can feel it between and sometimes below the testicles when erect. Figure 4, Additional Male Sweet Spots, on page 56 makes it clearer.

Most sexology literature tells us that the parts near vajra's head are the most excitable. We've confirmed that over and over. But Somraj has found that the base of his vajra produces a different kind of sensation when squeezed by a hand or pulsing sphincter. Since that only happens after about a half hour of play, you might not notice it during a quickie.

Though we haven't read about vajra's base being a distinct sweet spot elsewhere, the bulb is well documented. It makes sense that part of your erection is anchored inside. Otherwise your hard-on would just flop around. The bulb enjoys firm erotic touch between a man's testicles or just below them.

Vajra's Neighborhood

Those are a vajra's ten main erogenous zones. There are another ten in the neighborhood that often don't get enough sexual attention. These appear on figure 3, but figure 4 makes them clearer:

11. The *testicles* are the glands commonly called balls that hang below vajra's base.
12. The testicles are supported in a pouch called the *scrotum*.
13. The *perineum* is the region below the testicles and above the rosetta.

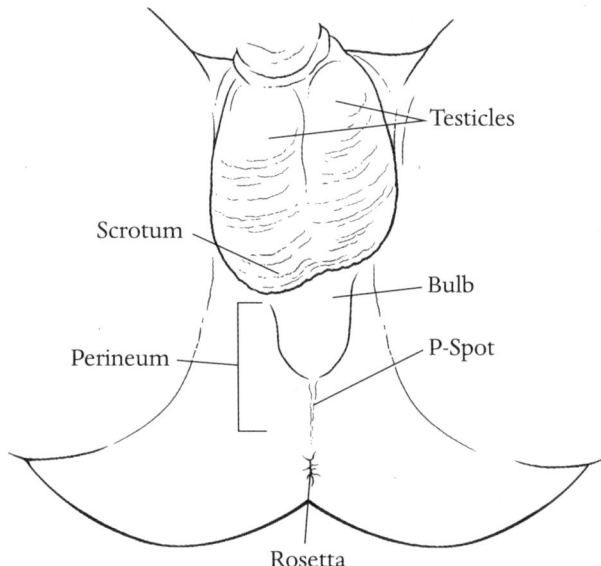

Figure 4: Additional Male Sweet Spots

14. The *P-spot* is a small, soft area of the perineum that you can find by feel more than by eye.
15. The *rosetta* is our name for the anus, the external opening at the bottom end of the gastrointestinal tract. This sensitive orifice of elimination between the butt cheeks is also loaded with nerve endings.

Pulling on a man's scrotum without bumping the glands inside is sometimes very arousing. Many, like Somraj, prefer a gentle caress, light scratching, or wet licking. In spite of their vulnerability, some men like more vigorous play with their scrotum and testicles.

Pushing into the P-spot, the soft tissue in the perineum below the testicles and bulb, is a way to stimulate a man's prostate gland from the outside. We prefer a more direct approach via the rosetta and the following inside sweet spots:

16. The *anal canal* is a one- to one-and-a-half-inch tube that extends inside from the rosetta. This channel is lined with soft, delicate mucous membranes and erectile cushions that contain a high concentration of tiny blood vessels and nerve endings.
17. The two *anal sphincters* in the canal keep it closed until needed.

18. The *rectum* is the lower part of the colon near the end of the gastrointestinal tract, which extends from the large intestine to the anal canal at the bottom.

With a little washing and attention to hygiene, backdoor sex that stimulates any or all of these erogenous zones can be highly exciting. Though these sweet spots are sensitive all by themselves, much of the excitement of male anal play stems from their close proximity to the prostate gland.

19. The *prostate gland* is an egg-shaped organ about the size of a chestnut or walnut. This firm, partly muscular gland is below the bladder and between it and the rectum.

The prostate has an unusual structure. It's composed of forty tiny mini-glands and ducts that secrete biochemicals. The little glands are surrounded by a muscular sheath that triggers ejaculation when it contracts. That's why the prostate is the control center for a man's ejaculatory orgasms.

We often call the prostate the *male G-spot* because the sensations resemble what happens to a woman during a G-spot climax. Though lots of sweet spots are potentially orgasmic, male G-spot play is something special.

20. The cross section of the *pelvic floor muscles* is shown in figure 3. If we had a muscle-sensitive X-ray machine, we'd be able to see the pelvic floor muscles under the skin snaking around the other organs in figure 4.

Though they're not really erogenous zones, we've included the bladder, above the prostate, and the coccyx, at the bottom of the spine, for orientation.

Vajra Erections

How does your vajra get erect? Getting engorged with blood is what makes it grow.

Vajra play causes blood to flow into the three spongy, cylindrical chambers. When the blood vessels around the base close off, the blood is trapped inside. That's what makes your member long and rigid. Anti-erectile-dysfunction medications do their magic by constricting those veins and capillaries.

Also, muscles in the vicinity get tighter and pull on vajra's head. This retracts your foreskin if you're uncircumcised. Erection also makes your scrotum thicken and contract so it becomes less baggy. Your testicles swell and elevate while your scrotum is pulled higher in toward your body.

Vasocongestion causes vajra's color to get deeper, redder, or even purple-headed. The pooling blood increases the warmth down there, spreading to your perineum. As you approach orgasm, your pelvic floor and anal muscles may begin to contract and spasm.

You may emit a few drops of *pre-come*, a clear fluid that's not semen. Still, it may contain some sperm. And, unless there's a finger inside your rosetta, you'll probably miss that your prostate gland enlarges with fluid.

Any part of a vajra can give pleasure when erect or not. We bet you've discovered that vajras can take a lot of vigorous exercise. Of course, there are limits, so be sure you don't rub vajra's skin raw without adequate lubrication or bend him too sharply.

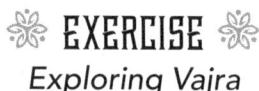

EXERCISE
Exploring Vajra

1. With a hand mirror, explore all the sweet spots on your vajra.
2. Play with your vajra and watch closely what happens and what you feel as it gets erect.
3. If you're both willing, let your partner do the same as you describe what you're feeling.

Summary and Action Steps

- A man's vajra has ten sweet spots (erogenous zones) plus ten more in the neighborhood.
- A vajra gets erect when its three spongy cylinders fill with blood.
- Learn more about vajra's sweet spots and erections with the Exploring Vajra Exercise.

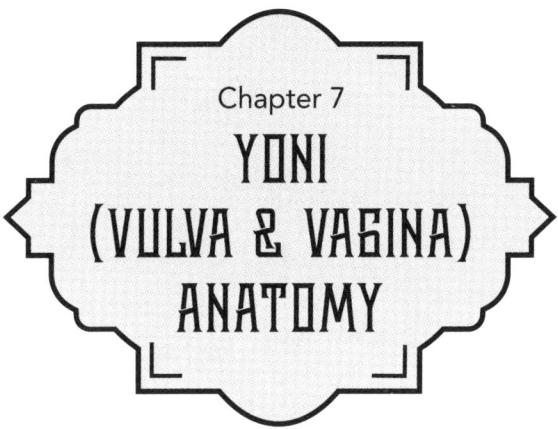

Chapter 7
YONI (VULVA & VAGINA) ANATOMY

No part of female anatomy has received so much attention, so much love, and so much abuse as the yoni. As you've seen, we use the Sanskrit word *yoni* instead of medical or street names. The outer yoni is the *vulva*, the part of the yoni that's visible when disrobed, and the inner yoni is the *vagina* or vaginal canal.

Yoni's Sweet Spots

There are thirty erogenous zones in and around a woman's yoni. First, we'll look at the twelve sweet spots on the outside. Figure 5, Closed Yoni Sweet Spots, on page 60 illustrates the following:

1. Pubic hair at the top of outer yoni covers the *mons*, *mons pubis*, or *mound of Venus*. This is a soft pad of tissue that rests over the top of a woman's pubic bone. Many women enjoy pressure on their mons. Some sex positions specialize in grinding the man's pelvic bone there.

Below the mons, a woman's yoni is protected by two soft vertical folds of skin that form a protective shield from the outside world when closed. We commonly call them lips though the official term is *labia*.

2. The *outer lips,* or *labia majora*, extend from the mound to below yoni's mouth. They are typically larger, longer, and fleshier than the inner lips. Most women have pubic hair that grows from the mound down the outer lips and sometimes on the inside, too.

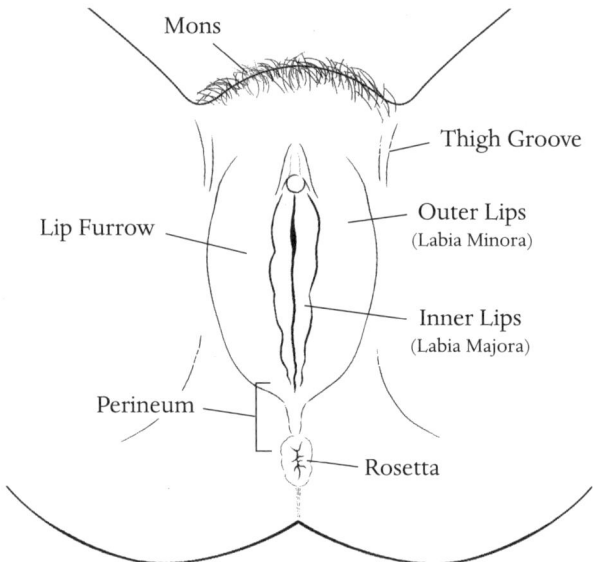

Figure 5: Closed Yoni Sweet Spots

3. Between the outer lips and the inner thighs are wide depressions we call the *thigh grooves*. They're fun to stroke and lick but not that sensitive.
4. The *inner lips,* or *labia minora,* are typically thinner and shorter than the outer lips and more sensitive. They surround and cover yoni's mouth before she's erect. Some women have longer inner lips that hang down. Whatever their form, they're all beautiful.
5. We call the sensitive crease between the inner and outer lips the *lip furrow.*
6. A woman's *rosetta* is the opening at the bottom of the gastrointestinal system.
7. On a woman's body, the *perineum* lies below outer yoni and above the rosetta.

Playing with the outer sweet spots is a good warmup during loveplay or fun any time.

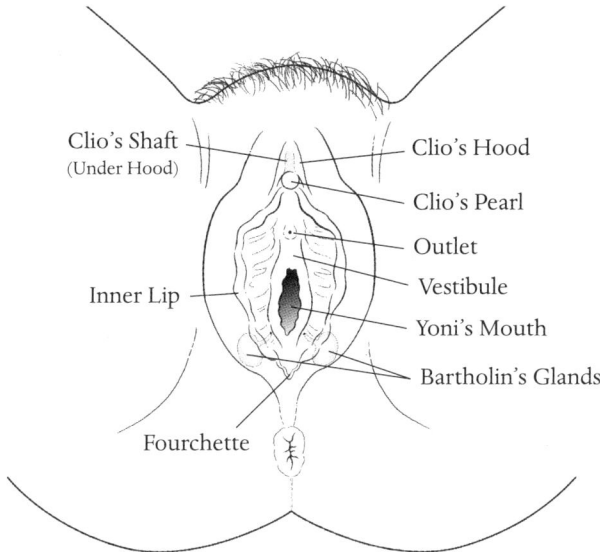

Figure 6: Spread Yoni Sweet Spots

When you spread a woman's inner lips, you'll expose even more highly responsive tissues as shown above in figure 6, Spread Yoni Sweet Spots:

8. The *vestibule* is the soft, tender tissue between the inner lips and above yoni's mouth. Jeffre really loves a moist fingerpad or tongue stroking here. The vestibule also contains the outlet of the urethra, which you'll see shortly.

9. *Yoni's mouth* is scientifically deemed the *vaginal introitus*. It's the soft, fleshy tissue around the opening to inner yoni. Around yoni's mouth are the inner lips, vestibule, and fourchette. The deeper you go, the more excitable the tissues become.

10. Yoni's mouth is surrounded by the *bulbospongiosus* muscle (previously called the *bulbocavernosus*), which functions like a vaginal sphincter. Because it's under the skin of the vestibule, it's not shown in figure 6 but will appear later.

11. The *fourchette* is a thick fold of skin at the bottom of the vestibule that surrounds the lower border of yoni's mouth.

12. The *Bartholin's glands* are two small pea-sized glands on either side of yoni's mouth that provide vaginal lubrication.

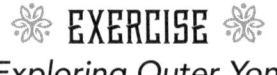 EXERCISE
Exploring Outer Yoni

1. With a hand mirror, explore all the sweet spots on the outside of your yoni.
2. Then do this exercise with your partner watching. Describe everything you're touching and how it feels.

Clio

At the top of the vestibule and below the mons is a woman's crown jewel, her *clio*. That's our name for the highly sensitive and erectile *clitoris*. This is the only human organ whose purpose is strictly dedicated to pleasure. Most women need some form of clio stimulation to orgasm.

Here are the clio's more visible components, which appear in figure 6:

13. Clio's *pearl* is the hypersensitive bud that, when erect, peeks out under a covering of skin at the apex where the inner lips meet. It's also known as the *glans*. Pearls vary considerably in size from woman to woman, though that doesn't appear to affect pleasure. Most are the size of a pea, a bit smaller than a rubber pencil eraser. After menopause, the clitoris can become over two times larger than it was during teenage years. Because of its proliferation of tiny blood vessels and eight thousand nerve endings, the pearl is a woman's most sensitive erogenous zone.

14. Clio's *hood* is small flap of fleshy tissue, quite thick on some women, that covers the pearl. If you pull back clio's hood, you may or may not see its pearl. Some clios aren't visible until they get erect and swell with excitement. Clio's hood is designed to protect the pearl from the friction of clothes and overstimulation during sexual play. These sensations can be intense, making them extremely uncomfortable. Too much stimulation too soon can be painful. The same occurs after an explosive orgasm.

15. Like vajras, clios also have a *shaft*, a loose cylinder of fibrous tissue, that heads upward about an inch toward a woman's belly under the hood and just below the mound of Venus. It's about the width of a lead pen-

cil and rests on top of a part of the pelvis referred to as the *pubic bone*. There's a cushion under clio's shaft and above this bone composed of a layer of fat and muscle. That's fortunate because most clios are so sensitive that this padding helps prevent overstimulation.

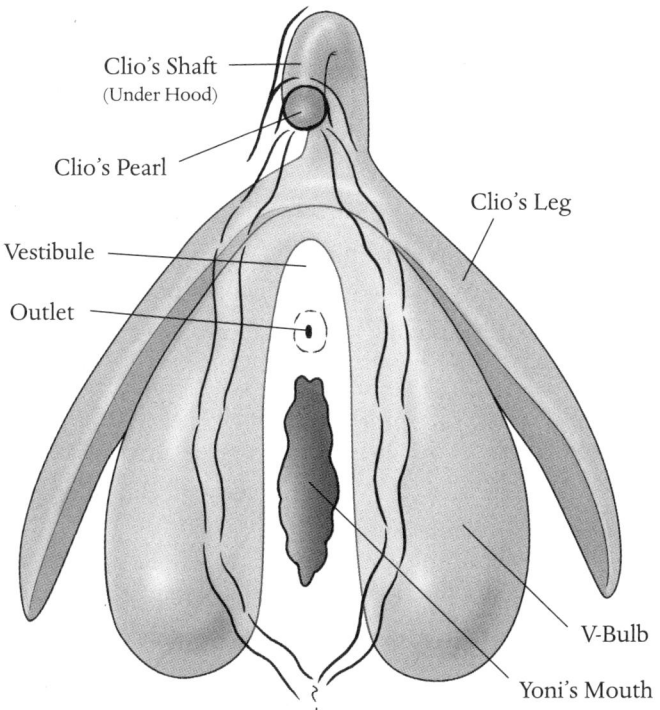

Figure 7: Inner Clio

The hood normally covers the pearl and shaft, which are often revealed when clio gets erect. But these two parts are only one quarter of clio's *corpus,* or *body,* which figure 7, Inner Clio, illustrates. The entire clio is about four inches long and has five parts, three-quarters of which are buried deep inside. And two of these deeper erectile parts have left and right lobes.

16. About an inch above the pearl, the top of clio's shaft bends down toward inner yoni. Then it forks into two *legs,* or *crura.* Clio's legs run along the lower part of the pubic bone and continue deeper inside for about three inches around either side of yoni's inner canal.

17. Clio's *vestibular bulbs,* or *V-bulbs,* are teardrop-shaped erectile lobes that lie on either side of yoni's mouth. They extend underneath the inner lips and beneath the vestibule. At the top, the V-bulbs are attached to clio's shaft. The V-bulbs and legs are made of the same kind of spongy tissue that fills with blood and makes jewel organs erect when aroused.

Inner Yoni's Sweet Spots

You probably know inner yoni as the *vagina*. It's a highly flexible muscular sheath from two and a half to four inches in length that extends inside from yoni's mouth. It's a deeply folded, ridged, expandable canal with a rich supply of nerves and blood vessels.

Inner yoni is lined with mucous membranes and is surrounded by erectile tissue. That means the surrounding walls fill with blood and get engorged just like a vajra. In fact, under desirable circumstances, inner yoni secretes lubrication and other liquids.

There are thirteen more sweet spots on a woman's body in and around her yoni that can contribute to her arousal and trigger orgasms. Figure 8, Inner Yoni, on page 65 is a side view that shows inner yoni and its erogenous zones alongside many of the previous ones.

18. A woman's *rectum* is the lower part of the colon.
19. The *anal canal* is the short tube extending inside from the rosetta into the rectum.
20. The two *anal sphincter*s surround the anal canal.
21. The *lower sponge* is an area of squishy erectile tissue beneath the perineum and between yoni's canal and the rectum. It's about one-half inch wide and usually lies one-half to one and a half inches inside. You can stimulate the lower sponge with a finger, tongue, vajra, or sex toy.

Yoni (Vulva & Vagina) Anatomy   65

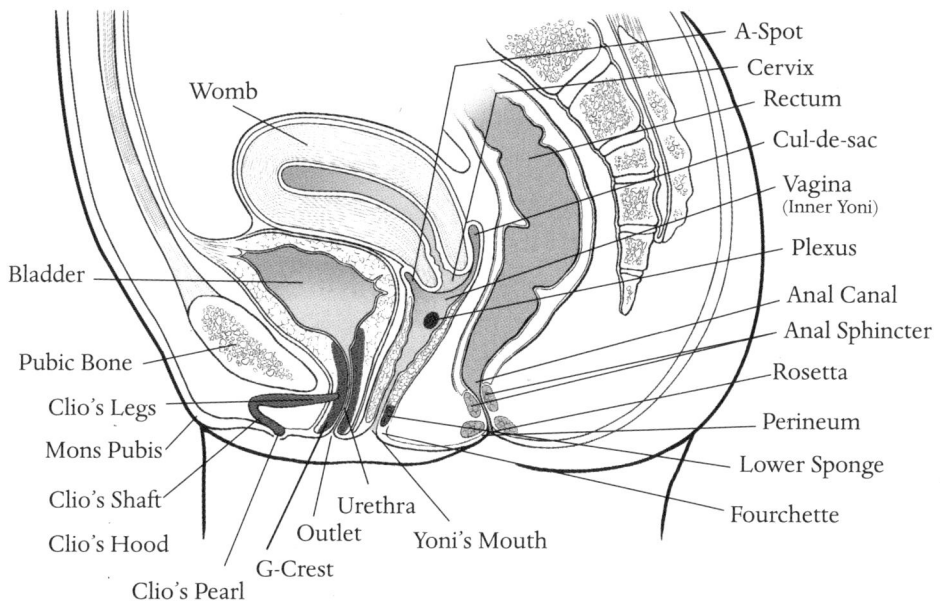

Figure 8: Inner Yoni

22. The *urethra* is the slender tube that transmits urine out of the body. It extends from the bladder to the outlet just above yoni's mouth.

23. The *outlet* is the opening of the urethral canal through which urine passes. It lies below a woman's clio within the inner lips and near the upper edge of yoni's mouth. In some women it's just inside yoni's mouth. The outlet is especially sensitive to sexual stimulation.

24. There's a rough, sensitive area inside yoni's canal on the upper front wall. Many experts tell you to look for this "secret orgasmic trigger," usually called the *G-spot*, one to two inches inside. This erogenous zone was named after Dr. Ernst Gräfenberg, a German gynecologist, who first published about it in 1950.

Actually, this area of spongy erogenous tissue isn't one clearly defined spot. It's the *urethral sponge* that surrounds the urethra from the outlet to the bladder. Because it protrudes downward into the canal when erect, we prefer to call this highly sensitive ridge the *G-crest*. Some sexologists believe the spongy erectile tissue connects to the clio's deeper lobes and the lower sponge.[4]

Some texts say that the G-crest feels like a hard bean under the surface. But our experience is that when arousal causes the spongy tissue to become engorged, it feels like corduroy.

We first experimented with finding the G-crest in our first Tantric sex workshop. Somraj stroked the upper wall of Jeffre's yoni with a finger curled back toward the heel of his palm in a come-hither gesture. As predicted, we found one rough, engorged area about an inch inside. As we continued the exercise, we found four more highly sensitive spots along the urethral sponge on inner yoni's upper wall and behind the pubic bone.

In fact, the female urethral sponge is populated with tiny glands analogous to the ones in the male prostate. Interestingly, they are distributed along the erectile sheath that surrounds the urethra in different locations in different women at different times. As a result, it appears that the sweet spots move based on which mini-glands are most engorged at that moment.

Deeper Yoni

Inner yoni's canal curves up from its mouth toward a woman's belly. Its outward third, the part closest to the mouth, is different in character than the inward two-thirds. The outer tissues are covered with ridges and furrows, especially around the urethral and lower sponges. Because it's dense with nerve endings, the walls of the outer portion are highly responsive to touch and friction.

The deeper two-thirds of inner yoni have smoother walls with fewer nerve endings. Consequently, this inner area responds less to touch and more to the kind of pressure produced from a firm rod of flesh, plastic, or rubber. Here are the sweet spots farther inside shown in figure 8:

25. The *plexi* are two intricate braided nerve bundles located deep on either side of inner yoni's canal. Each plexus is highly sensitive when prodded.
26. The *uterus* or *womb* is a hollow muscular organ, shaped like an upside-down pear, that lies between the bladder and rectum above inner yoni and the pubic bone.

---

4. Somraj Pokras and Jeffre TallTrees, *Female Ejaculation* (Berkeley, CA: Amorata/Ulysses Press, 2009).

27. The *cervix* is the tiny muscular passageway at the top end of yoni's canal. This is the entrance to the womb. Except during childbirth, the cervix is quite narrow, maybe the size of the tip of a ballpoint pen. Some sexologists believe that thrusting against the womb or cervix can trigger a deep resounding orgasm. Not all women like this though.

Figure 8 shows some space inside inner yoni. At rest, yoni's mouth is closed, and the sides of the canal are collapsed upon themselves. That leaves no space between the walls when they're touching each other. But you know the inner yoni can stretch enough to accommodate an erection and even farther for a baby.

A little-appreciated fact of the yoni's geography is the open triangle at the top. You'll notice little crevices above and below the cervix. Each is called a *fornix*, the technical name for a little cleft or open-ended pouch, derived from *arch* in Latin.

28. The *A-spot,* or *anterior fornix,* on the belly side is very close to a woman's bladder. Prodding it can lead to rapid vaginal lubrication, ejaculation, and orgasm.
29. The posterior one (toward the back) has the cute name *cul-de-sac.* It's known to generate deep uterine orgasms when rammed with vajra's head or a dildo.
30. Various levels of a woman's *pelvic floor muscles* intertwine around yoni's mouth and her rosetta. They don't appear in figure 8 but will in a later figure.

For orientation, figure 8 also shows the pubic bone and bladder, though they're not really erogenous zones.

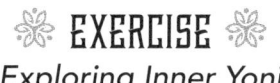

EXERCISE
Exploring Inner Yoni

1. With your fingers, explore all the sweet spots inside your yoni that you can reach.
2. Next, use a dildo to find the deeper ones.

3. Then do this exercise with your partner watching as you describe what you're feeling.
4. Finally let them explore inside your yoni themselves.

Yoni Erection

A full yoni erection is as essential for a woman as a vajra erection is to a man. Jewel union isn't particularly pleasant or exciting for a woman without full arousal. Far less than half of women can orgasm from a stroking vajra alone.

Regrettably, yoni erections are less obvious than vajra ones. Like men, when a woman is aroused, her metabolism, respiration, heart rate, blood pressure, hormone release, nerve traffic, and sex flush increase. Muscle tension typically causes a woman's nostrils to flare, her breasts to swell, and her nipples to harden. As a result, everything gets more sensitive.

But how does her yoni change? Yoni erections are caused by the spongy erectile tissues in and around the jewels filling with blood and becoming engorged. This tumescence makes the outer lips spread and flatten. The inner lips swell, lengthen, thicken, and darken. Clio's hood, the vestibule, and the fourchette turn redder.

At the same time, yoni's mouth and the perineum get plumper. The G-crest bulges downward, the V-bulbs expand, clio's legs stiffen, and the lower sponge swells, all pressing into inner yoni's canal. The large muscles surrounding yoni's mouth stretch and widen.

The clio swells with blood, which causes it to enlarge, lengthen, and puff up. The hood darkens in color and smooths out. As the pearl widens and gets firmer, it might stick out like a little erect vajra. Clio's shaft also expands and gets more rigid, almost like a thick, taut cable. The bend at the top of clio's shaft flattens a bit. That rotates clio's pearl outward so it emerges from under the hood.

These dramatic changes to outer yoni form a *puffy cuff*.[5] This is a snug, swollen, sensitive sleeve that surrounds and squeezes anything that's inserted. This soft, springy cushion is an integrated matrix of linked, excitable, erogenous zones on all sides of yoni's outer regions.

---

5. Sheri Winston, *Women's Anatomy of Arousal* (Kingston, NY: Mango Garden Press, 2010), chap. 6.

The cuff encompasses the outer and inner lips; yoni's mouth; clio's pearl, shaft, and legs; the V-bulbs; the G-crest; and the lower sponge. Though elastic, this puffy cuff is firmer and much "grabbier" than an unaroused yoni. This increases the friction around a vajra's in-stroke and grasps firmly on the out-stroke.

From the outside, all of this makes an engorged yoni appear like a blooming pink flower.

As orgasm approaches, a woman's clio swells and reddens further. The pearl retracts inward hiding under the hood again. Inner yoni's walls thicken, darken in color, and get more sensitive. The muscles that surround the canal contract and tighten, especially around yoni's mouth. While all this is happening, the womb enlarges, lifts up, and rotates forward. This lengthens yoni's canal. Vasocongestion and the changes to the uterus cause the deeper two-thirds of the canal to lengthen, expand, and open. At the same time, the outer third tends to tighten and contract.

This expansion of the open upper triangle around the cervix is called *yoni tenting*. The tenting effect causes a sucking pressure, presumably to draw sperm ups toward the womb.

The lifting and tilting of the womb causes the cervix to tilt back and draw upward. This retraction of the cervix also exposes the plexi, the pelvic nerve bundles on either side of deep yoni's canal. All this makes powerful thrusting more pleasurable.

Increased blood circulation causes the mucous membranes that line yoni's walls to secrete a clear, slick fluid. There's also a thick, slippery fluid that comes from the little Bartholin's glands. When a young woman is aroused, there's a good chance, but not 100 percent, that she will naturally produce this lubrication.

When super excited, some women ejaculate a clear fluid that we call *amrita*, the Sanskrit word for the goddesses' nectar of life. Though female ejaculation usually occurs during a form of orgasm, it offers a unique kind of peak pleasure.

❊ EXERCISE ❊
Yoni Erection

1. Self-pleasure outer yoni until your erection grows. As your puffy cuff forms, notice how your lips and clio change.
2. Next, do the same inside yoni, feeling how your lower sponge and G-crest grow.
3. Use a dildo to stimulate your plexi, cervix, and deep fornices.
4. Then do this exercise with your partner watching as you describe what you're feeling.
5. If you're willing, let your partner try what you've demonstrated.

Summary and Action Steps

- There are twelve outer yoni sweet spots you can see when a woman spreads her legs.
- Use the Exploring Outer Yoni Exercise to find a woman's outer sweet spots.
- The clio has five sweet spots, some of which extend deeper around the yoni.
- Inner yoni's sweet spots include the G-crest or urethral sponge, which is much more than one well-defined spot.
- Use the Exploring Inner Yoni Exercise to find a woman's thirteen inner sweet spots.
- Use the Yoni Erection Exercise to fully appreciate the color, puffiness, and feel of a woman's full erection.

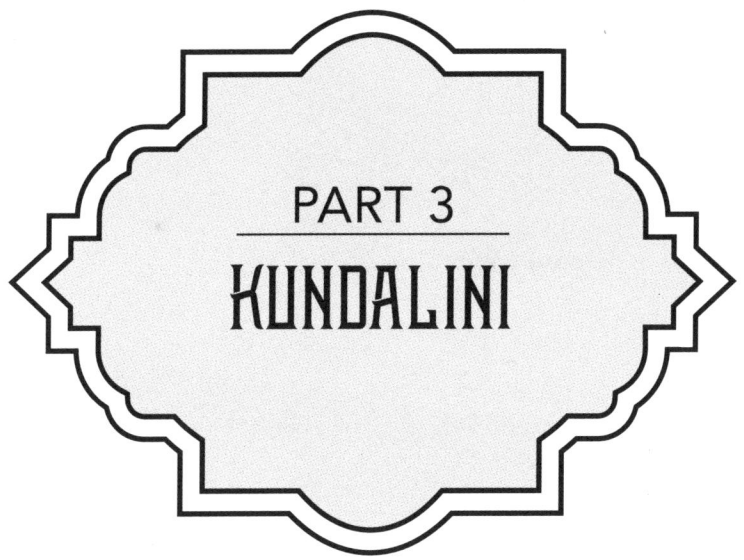

PART 3
KUNDALINI

We're confident the previous tour of male and female sweet spots will come in handy as we look into amplifying kundalini during penetration in this part and the next.

PART 3 will help you understand what kundalini does as it streams through your body. We'll introduce you to some potent energy practices to direct these currents and consciously magnify your passion. That includes running and streaming energy, filling your pleasure balloon, using the chakras, amplifying ecstasy, toning your sexual muscles, and breathing orgasmically.

Or, as so many of our teachers have said, just follow the energy, baby.

Chapter 8
ENERGY

What causes goose bumps? A chill down your spine? Shivers or ticklishness? Or how about that warm, tingly feeling in your jewels when you see a juicy specimen of your preferred gender? Or that phenomenal shaking that wracks your body when you come?

This is kundalini at work. Are you aware of these ever-present vibrations inside? Can you feel them now? After years of practice, we feel them whenever we touch. And most times when we sit in silent meditation.

The term *energy* means the nervous and physical excitation that causes these feelings. It's the subtle inner pulsation that's always percolating beneath your normal level of consciousness.

In China it's called *chi*, in India it's called *prana*, in Japan it's called *ki*, in yoga it's called *kundalini*, but it's all energy. We're talking about the same electrical and magnetic universal lifeforce that pervades and animates your body. It's the source of the pleasure you can generate in your body with the right kind of stimulation.

All matter, including all parts of your body, is in motion and radiating energy. Your cells, your blood, and your nerves all vibrate continuously.

You might not notice kundalini moving within. That's probably because it's a higher finer frequency than your internal receiver is tuned to. But you can train yourself to be more sensitive to subtle sexual energy flows.

We did. Somraj still remembers when our first Tantra teacher, Margot Anand, would talk about kundalini in front of the class. The teaching assistants on either side of her would shiver from just hearing about it. Somraj couldn't share that experience then, but he can now. So can you.

Dancing with Kundalini

From the moment your love and lust begin to charge the space around you, you are dancing with kundalini. You are generating and responding to sexual and orgasmic energy.

The instant your eyes meet, you may feel tingling inside. Your hearts may flutter and your jewels may stir. Initiating a date, creating a sacred space, discussing the partnering questions, exchanging sweet everythings, sharing loveplay—all these things activate energy at different chakras.

Awakened kundalini makes touching electric. Deep, wet kissing sends chills and shivers throughout your beings. A vajra's first contact with a yoni or rosetta can be earth-shattering. Focusing on sweet spots during jewel union galvanizes your circuits with passion.

If you stay fully connected, the merger of your energies can sweep you away into an altered space and another dimension.

Different Experiences of Kundalini

Everyone experiences kundalini a bit differently. In her great book *Women's Anatomy of Arousal*, Sheri Winston explains, "Some people experience sexual energy as moving heat, like a flow of molten lava or a torrent of hot water. Others feel vibrations pulsing through them. Some see light and colors swirling. People sometimes report sounds thrumming and beating rhythms inside them. Some feel sensations tingling and awakening various body parts. Yet others report multiple sensations that mutate as the energy awakens, builds and surges about."[6]

Learning to make love on multiple levels of body, heart, mind, and soul begins by increasing your sensitivity to the sensations of kundalini. Your "radio receiver" needs to be tuned to this finer frequency in whatever way works for you.

After some reading, Jeffre learned to discern energy by making a conscious choice to become more mindful of its sensations. Trained as a chemist, it was harder for Somraj. But when he embraced the Tantric attitude and shifted his

---

6. Sheri Winston, *Women's Anatomy of Arousal* (Kingston, NY: Mango Garden Press, 2010), chap. 11.

attention to his body, he began to notice the subtleties of kundalini fermenting within. Gradually we could both feel blossoms of sexual energy inside.

Do you get that sexual energy is often subtle at first yet powerful when you harness it? It often starts as a trickling spring before it fountains into a powerful tidal wave that sweeps you away.

Building Your Kundalini

You need to build your kundalini to fully enjoy Supernatural Sex. Because sexual energy is in part fire, it needs the heat of an excited body. It needs a spark from attraction, desire, lust, love, or other strong emotions. It needs oxygen from deep breathing. It needs the fuel of your lifeforce.

Because sexual energy is also electricity, touch and movement activate it. Sexual biochemistry and pheromones, spurred by taste and smell, add to it. The right words, memory, sext, image, or email can kindle it. Sometimes just your honey's appearance fans the flames. You can use your imagination to create the fuel through visualization.

During jewel union you target sweet spots and tap into their pools of pleasure to fill your body to the brim with kundalini. You make love as long as you can. You keep the fire burning hot and the current charging higher and higher.

In ordinary sex, when you contact a sexually charged stream, you go for it. Unfortunately, an explosive climax can end your playtime prematurely. The energy you've been building is released, and you have to wait to recharge your batteries.

Climaxes are wonderful when you've had your fill, but they can't compare to the lasting heights you can create by playing in the Valley for one or more hours. If you want to experience all the joys of Supernatural Sex, you'll need to build and conserve kundalini, not lose it. The big question is how to keep it from dissipating when you're riding the waves to higher and higher peaks.

Biofield

Building kundalini charges your biofield, which we previously talked about in chapter 2, Energy Tools, when we introduced the pleasure balloon (see figure 2 on page 20). Your biomagnetic force field is a luminous, multicolored, cocoon encircling you up and down, left and right, front and back. This egg-shaped energy reservoir conducts glowing streamers of bioelectricity, which make the air inside it shimmer and tingle.

The more aroused you get, the more energy your biofield contains. And when you feel close intimacy, heart-connection, and soul merger, you welcome another into your biofield. Biofield fusion partly explains why we love jewel union so much. So many points of contact connect multiple sweet spots with energetic channels.

The more kundalini you generate and pump into your pleasure balloon, the bigger it gets. It expands up your chakras way past your jewels and inflates to fill your whole body and the biofield around it.

Which means ecstatic vibrations will spread all over your body. Which means you'll feel like you're floating away on a cloud of ecstasy. Since you're not wasting that juicy lifeforce, you can do it over and over. This is a little glimpse into the rarified stratosphere of energy orgasm.

How to Fill Your Pleasure Balloon

The Tantric attitude is essential to fill your pleasure balloon gradually. Feel the sensations in your body. Let them be and relax into them. Go slow and allow your arousal to climb at its own rate. Stretch this elastic container in small steps so you can contain more energy without tensing up.

How you manage the expansion and contraction of your energy sac is what regulates how much pleasure you feel at each point. If you're out of shape sexually and your balloon is brittle from lack of exercise, you won't be able to absorb as much pleasure. If it's restricted to the small area of your jewels, it could expand too rapidly and pop.

The more you exercise your bubble, the more flexible it becomes, the easier it expands, and the larger it can get. The old maxim "use it or lose it" applies here. Without regular sexual practice, whether solo or partnered, the walls of your pleasure balloon shrink and become stiff. The energy channels that fill the bubble clog and close.

With a fully inflated pleasure balloon, you have much more sexual electricity to play with. You can funnel it back into your sweet spots to make them more sensitive. You can use it to recharge your jewels if they get a bit depleted before you're done.

Full-body orgasm happens when you fill your biofield to the brim with this bristling lifeforce. And when you go for the Big O, it can supercharge your climax into a cosmic explosion.

When your lover is doing the same, your biofields can merge. If you've ever felt one with your beloved while making love, you know what we mean.

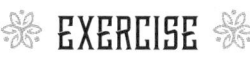

EXERCISE

Pleasure Balloon

1. Sit still with your eyes closed and watch your breath move in and out.
2. After your mind stills, notice which sensations you feel everywhere in your body. Take a moment to register each separately.
3. Touch yourself softly all over and keep watching inside. Notice where your sensations grow.
4. Then concentrate on your jewels. As you touch your jewels, notice where your kundalini is percolating, moving, and pooling.
5. If you relax into it, you should be able to feel your pleasure balloon buzz and pulse. Take your time pleasuring yourself and use your intention to see if you can make it expand and fill your biofield.

Directing Your Energy

When there's enough energy in your pleasure balloon, you can consciously direct where it goes. Somraj runs energy to his vajra if his erection is waning. Jeffre runs energy to sweet spots inside her yoni to trigger bigger orgasms.

Raising kundalini from its dormant seat around your jewels is fundamental to expanding your pleasure balloon. Then you can direct it to your heart to enhance intimacy, to your mind for clearer vision, and to your soul to energize your connection with the Divine.

When your pleasure balloon is full and energy runs freely through your channels, it tends to stream of its own accord.

We celebrate how much we love the sexual friction of jewel union. But when our pleasure balloons are so vitalized that we're both throbbing all over with love and passion, something supernatural happens.

Summary and Action Steps

- Learn to increase your sensitivity to orgasmic energy.
- Make love as long as you can to fill your body with kundalini.
- Use the Pleasure Balloon Exercise to become more aware of your energy bubble.
- Fill your pleasure balloon slowly until it fully inhabits your biofield.

Chapter 9
CHANNELS

Your body is alive with all kinds of bioenergy. As a result, your senses, nerves, glands, muscles, blood, lungs, and cells are in constant motion. It's your lifeforce that animates all these processes.

Kundalini is another facet of this power, albeit at first glance a subtler one. In chapter 2, Energy Tools, we defined it as the electromagnetic lifeforce responsible for libido, pleasure, and orgasm. In simpler terms, it's just sexual energy.

Sexual energy can lie dormant everywhere, asleep in hidden reservoirs or pools. You might feel it, but it doesn't impact you much unless it's moving.

You should be able to feel a slight current if you relax, empty your mind, and put the palms of your hands or the soles of your feet together. As you become more adept at channeling energy, you'll become more sensitized to your own unique electromagnetic pathways.

To take full advantage of your kundalini, you need to increase your awareness of the conduits in which sexual energy flows. We all have physiological circuits like nerves that electrical impulses follow. Kundalini tends to run along subtler channels of the sort that acupuncturists address. The ancients called these subtle energy conduits *nadis*.

Chakras

Learning to channel kundalini begins by heightening your awareness of your chakras. We've already discussed these energy centers briefly, but we'd like to go more in-depth. The *chakras*, the Indian word for spinning wheels, are seven energy centers that govern different types of body electricity, human magnetism, and lifeforce. They are arrayed from the bottom of your pelvis to the top of your head.

These seven vortices are like invisible whirlpools loosely connected to your spine. They function something like electrical transformers that link your physical body to your energy body and soul.

Chakras are where different qualities of lifeforce energy are generated, collected, and transmitted, like sexual energy, self-image, and higher wisdom.

The seven chakras shown in figure 9 on page 81 are as follows:

#	Chakra	Location
1st	Root	Base of the spine or pelvic floor
2nd	Belly	Two inches below navel
3rd	Solar Plexus	Below the breast bone
4th	Heart	Center of the chest
5th	Throat	Throat
6th	Third Eye	Forehead
7th	Crown	Top of the head

Though energy is energy, when it's active in one chakra, it feels different from the others. The first or root chakra regulates reproduction and physical survival. The sex drive here is biological like animal lust. The second chakra deals with the body and its emotions. The sensations of moving energy in Supernatural Sex stem from the belly chakra.

The third chakra, the solar plexus, manages personal power and identity. At the fourth, the heart chakra, you perceive this lifeforce as the warm embrace of love. Your voice, values, and beliefs underlying your truth emanate from the throat chakra, number five. The sixth chakra is the third eye. Here is where your intuition fuels your vision and higher awareness. The crown or seventh chakra connects you to the wisdom of the spiritual plane.

Tantric attitude exercises like meditating, creating a sacred space, and the partnering questions are designed to activate different chakras. To get friendlier with your chakras, tune your awareness with the Chakra Breathing Exercise.

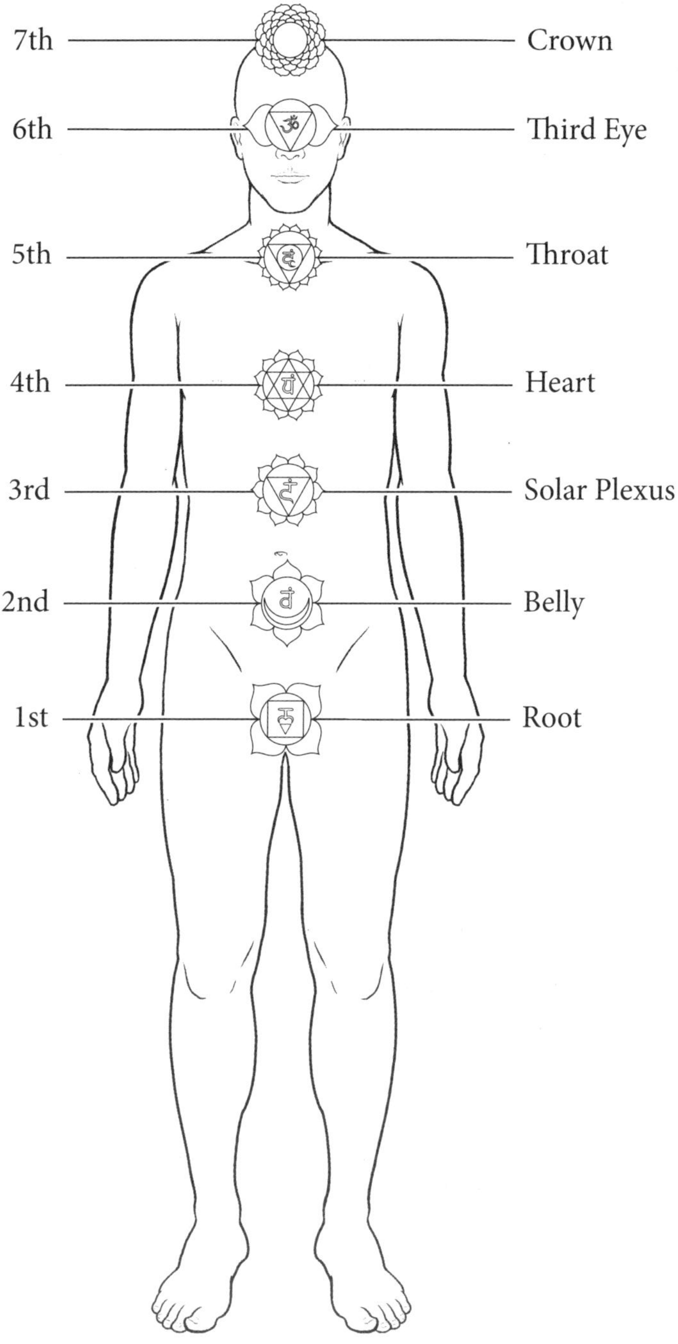

Figure 9: Chakras

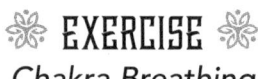
EXERCISE
Chakra Breathing

1. Sit in meditation until you feel centered and grounded.
2. Imagine each breath flowing in and out of your first chakra for a few minutes.
3. Notice any sensations that emerge as your breath cleanses and charges your first chakra.
4. Repeat this at the second chakra.
5. Do the same at each chakra as you work your way up to the top of your head.
6. Focus on sensations anywhere in your body that cleansing and charging your chakras bring up.

Since you'll be working with subtle energy, you may need to repeat this exercise quite a few times until you can sense each spinning vortex.

Engaging the Chakras in Lovemaking

How does awakening your chakras help your sex life? The simple answer is that your chakras contain and control all the energies that come into play during lovemaking. Cleanse, charge, and connect your chakras and you can reach new heights of sensation, emotion, love, understanding, sensitivity, pleasure, and ecstasy.

Engaging different chakras by placing your attention on them adds a magical quality to otherwise ordinary sex. Start by mastering your sexual anatomy and arousal pathways (first chakra). When your jewels are coupled, revel in your lust and primal urges.

Get in your body and heighten your senses with Tantric touch and sensual massage. Let orgasmic energy fill your body with sensations of pleasure that spark between you (second chakra).

Stay present, secure, and grounded as you show up fully, and reveal your true self. Take responsibility for your own pleasure and guide your lovemaking to meet your own desires. Accept and respect your beloved without games, secrets, manipulation, or power trips (third chakra).

Use eye-gazing and intimacy-bonding rituals to activate heart energy. Shower your honey with affection and sweet everythings. Surrender yourself to love as you're consumed with compassion and appreciation (fourth chakra).

Recognize your values and beliefs. Openly share your thoughts and feelings. Speak your truth and hold nothing back. Ask for everything you want (fifth chakra).

The lifeforces released by your lovemaking energize your brain, mind, and sixth sense. Adopt an elevated conscious viewpoint, witness everything that happens, and let intuition guide you (sixth chakra).

Meditate together to open your crown to the heavens. Experience no soul separation between each other and with the Divine (seventh chakra).

Supernatural Sex aims to create an all-chakra connection where your seven centers all fire. You might compare it to a rainbow of different-hued orgasms happening throughout your body at the same time.

Opening Energy Channels

The more you work with your chakras, the easier it will be to run and stream energy. Routine practice will increase your sensitivity to the kundalini channels in your physical and energy bodies.

The most fundamental nadi is the *inner flute*, the conduit that connects your seven chakras, shown in figure 10 on page 84. Your inner flute extends from the base of your pelvis to the top of your head. Put one hand above and one below and see what you can sense right now. Though the inner flute isn't a physical organ, it's very real and extremely useful for channeling kundalini.[7]

There are other energy pathways as well. Later we'll explain how to open other circuits that connect your sweet spots and charge other parts of your body.

If there are blocks in the connections between the chakras, kundalini won't be able to fully flow through your inner flute and fill your pleasure balloon. A vital step in mastering Supernatural Sex is to open the linkages between pairs of adjacent chakras. Focused breathing can accelerate clearing those pathways so subtle energy can flow more smoothly.

---

7. Margot Anand, *The Art of Sexual Ecstasy* (Los Angeles: Tarcher, 1989), 163–168.

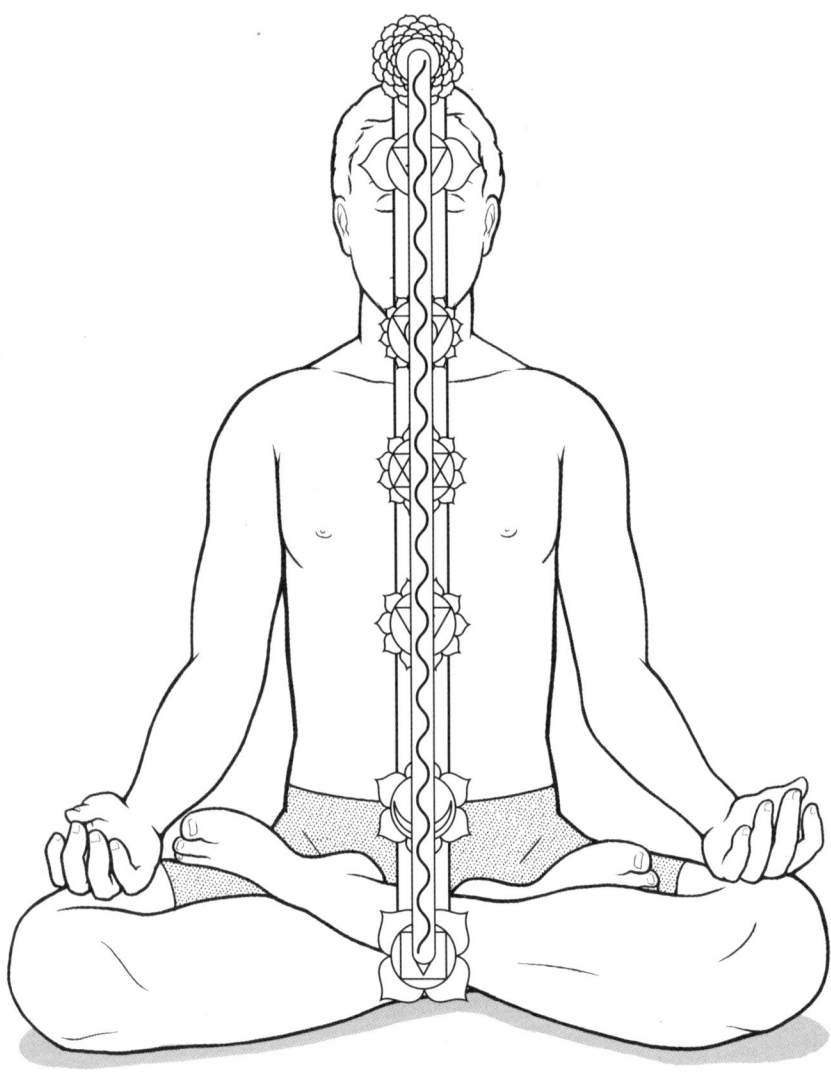

Figure 10: Inner Flute

❋ EXERCISE ❋
Inner Flute

1. Once you have a handle on breathing in and out of each chakra, focus on the linkages between them.
2. To start, breathe into the first chakra. Visualize the energy flowing up to the second on the in-breath. On the out-breath, imagine the charge settling back to the first chakra and then out of your body.
3. Repeat this for each pair of energy centers to cleanse the channels. Gradually you will feel the links in your inner flute opening more fully.

Summary and Action Steps

- Become more aware of kundalini flows in your nadis.
- Sit in meditation with your palms or soles of your feet together to sense kundalini.
- Heighten your awareness of your chakras using the Chakra Breathing Exercise.
- Engage all your chakras when you make love.
- Open the linkages between your chakras with the Inner Flute Exercise.

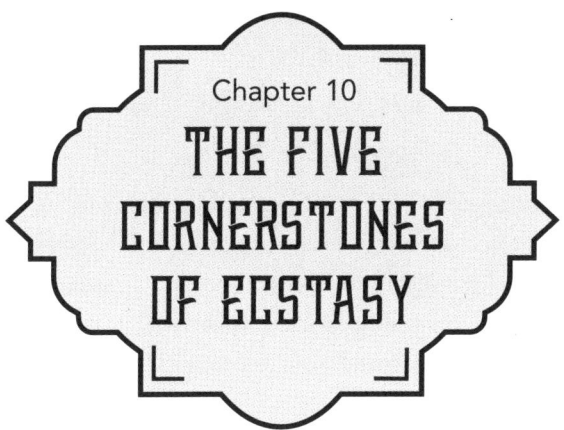

Chapter 10
THE FIVE CORNERSTONES OF ECSTASY

The more you tune in to sexual energy, the easier you can channel it up your inner flute and fill your pleasure balloon. This is how you create supernatural levels of ecstasy.

Ecstasy is the overwhelming feeling of excitement, joy, delight, and elated bliss that produces a trancelike state of euphoric rapture. It's an extraordinary elevation of the soul so intense that you're carried away beyond the reach of rational thoughts and ordinary impressions. It happens when you're filled with overwhelming emotion or overpowering energy that spills over your normal borders.

Supernatural Sex uses the five natural human responses to arousal to heighten ecstasy. You can turn these orgasmic reactions into simple tools to willfully expand your pleasure.

What happens when you approach orgasm? Your focus narrows, you breathe deeper and faster, you make noise, you move sensuously, and you see fireworks exploding around you. This is what passion looks like and what ecstasy feels like.

We call these inherent responses the *five cornerstones of ecstasy*:

1. **Being Present:** being relaxed and conscious in the present moment
2. **Tantric Breath:** using the intake and release of air through your mouth to energize you
3. **Love Sounds:** harnessing the power of your voice to stimulate energy flow

4. **Erotic Movement:** moving your body sensuously and using your sexual muscles to pump energy

5. **Visualization:** creating an image in your mind's eye of what you want to feel

When you consciously harness these natural orgasmic reactions, you can magnify your turn-on by choice. There are good and bad ways to use the five cornerstones. If you panted hysterically, tuned out, mumbled nonsense, and tensed up, these elements might block your kundalini flow. When you direct these natural responses to expand your sensations, you'll find your sensitivity and capacity for pleasure increase.

1. Being Present

Being present means showing up fully, mind, body, and soul. The first cornerstone, *presence*, is just another word for consciousness. Consequently, it has more to do with the third eye or sixth chakra.

To be present means to be completely aware—psychologically, emotionally, physically, and spiritually—of what's happening both inside and out. It's all of you here, now. Presence also implies a state of inner peace and mental stillness, which the Tantric attitude fosters.

Too often the monkey-mind busily chatters away with nonessentials that keep us from really feeling or being. Do you know the joke about the woman who "beiges out"? She's lying on her back while her husband is making love to her and she says, "This ceiling would look great painted beige."

Being fully present means being relaxed enough to open your senses in the moment without any goal or expectation. Sink into your sensations and feelings. Focus totally on the pleasure you receive right now.

To move into those higher states of awareness where ecstasy lies, it's essential to leave the mundane world behind. You can develop the cornerstone of presence by practicing staying in the moment, feeling your body, and clearing your mind. Practicing meditation can help you be more present in your body and out of your head.

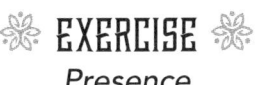
Presence

1. Repeat the Conscious Breathing Exercise from chapter 3 about the Tantric attitude.
2. Once you settle in, open your awareness as wide as you can to everything that's happening inside and out.
3. Simply focus on the here and now.

2. Tantric Breath

The average person inhales only one pint of air while fully expanded lungs can hold seven. The more air you take in, the more you can increase your erotic charge.

The second cornerstone, the *Tantric breath*, is slow, through the mouth, and deep into the belly. It fills your lungs more fully and feeds your sexual fire. You can turn yourself on with the Tantric breath alone. If you breathe this way when you're already excited, you will wash yourself inside and out with kundalini. That allows you to get higher for longer.

Breathing this way increases your sensitivity. Just imagining your breath fully penetrating a limb, gland, or organ brings sensations of warmth and aliveness. It's like touching yourself from the inside. The Tantric breath is a powerful sexual tool you can use to heighten your arousal, relax yourself, and regulate your excitement.

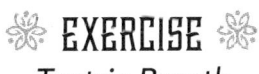
Tantric Breath

1. Sit comfortably, close your eyes, and focus on your normal breathing.
2. Breathe through your mouth and gradually increase your intake of air. Go as slowly as you can while remaining comfortable.
3. See how much air you can take in if you push yourself to the limit.
4. Once you've found that place, back off until you can breathe deeply without any strain.

3. Love Sounds

Supernatural Sex is loud and noisy. Making erotic *love sounds*, the third cornerstone, broadcasts the pleasure you're feeling. Vocalizing releases inhibitions, opens nerve channels, and stimulates kundalini flow.

We cry out a lot when we're turned-on. Jeffre shrieks, Somraj growls, and we both moan and bellow. Plus, you can hear us shouting "Yes," "Wow!" and "Oh my God!"

Sound moves energy beyond your jewels and disperses it throughout your body to all your cells. Making sensuous sounds causes vibrations that resonate with your kundalini, which amplifies your ecstasy. Sometimes your tissues and organs need you to express their primal power with grunts and squeals.

The same nerves that regulate your voice box are connected to your jewels. This cornerstone is regulated by your fifth or throat chakra. If you're quiet during lovemaking, it's probably somewhat closed. This can limit your ability to be clear and ask for what you want.

We recommend you make a genuine effort to open your throat. Making gut-level noises can release pent-up energy that could block your flow of pleasure. Start by sincerely embracing the Tantric attitude. Be present, immerse yourself in sensations, and turn them into expressive sounds.

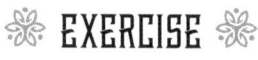 EXERCISE
Love Sounds

1. To practice, sit comfortably and start the Tantric breath.
2. As you exhale, make the sound "ahhhh."
3. Practice using the vowels: a, e, i, o, and u.
4. Next, try it while you're self-pleasuring. Vibrate your throat with different guttural sounds to see which one most intensifies your pleasure and spreads it through your body.
5. Agree during the partnering questions to practice the next time you make love.
6. As his vajra thrusts in, both exhale and say "ooo" as loud as you can muster. As his vajra withdraws, inhale and say "ahhh" as forcefully as you can in your voice box.

Don't you find that hearing your playmate wail, shout, and bellow adds an erotic boost? If your sexual voice is restrained, you might ask your partner if your moans and groans of pleasure are a turn-on.

Of course, with shallow breathing you won't have much air to make sounds with. That's why the Tantric breath and making love sounds work closely together.

4. Erotic Movement

We don't have to explain why jewel union requires pelvic rocking. Isn't it hotter when the receiver pushes back to meet your strokes? A turned-on body can't help but move erotically. Inhibited lovers suppress those movements.

When we approach orgasm, the shocks of kundalini igniting inside make our nerves fire and our muscles spasm. The surging energy causes Somraj to shimmy, shudder, and shake. At a pleasure peak, Jeffre writhes, rocks, and jerks. Our arms and legs flail, our bodies undulate like a snake, and sometimes we jackknife uncontrollably.

Streaming kundalini often shows up as one or a series of *kriyas*. Kriyas are involuntary, spontaneous twitches, jerks, or jolts of the body in response to moving energy. They often morph into delightful shaking.

You can intentionally use the *erotic movement* cornerstone to run energy. Your body has its own erotic rhythm and knows how to respond to pleasure if you let it. Watch an exotic dancer or an Elvis Presley performance and you'll know what we mean.

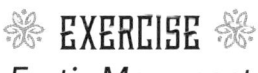
Erotic Movement

1. Use erotic movement to amplify your turn-on. If you're tight, start with some yoga or pelvic stretching.
2. Play some rhythmic music. Stand with your knees slightly bent and rock your hips in time with the beat.
3. The next time you make love, arrange yourselves in sex positions that allow you both to dance with your sexual thrusts.

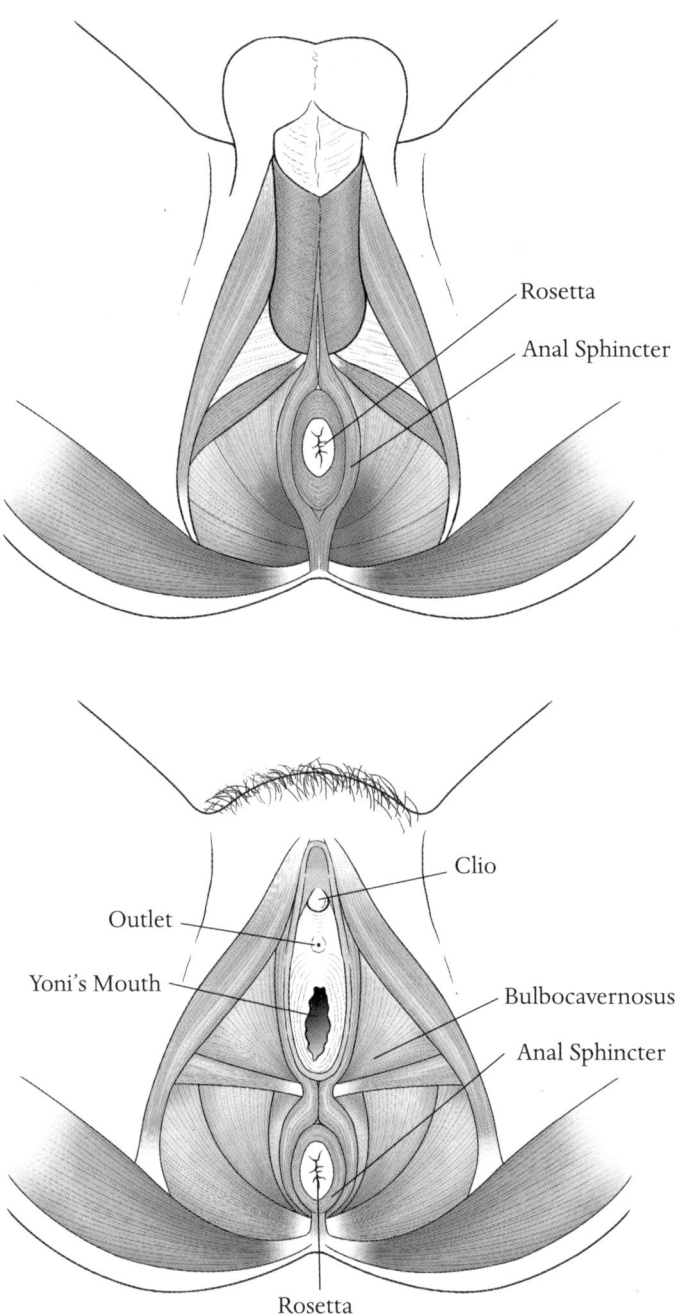

Figure 11: Pelvic Floor Muscles

Sexual Muscles

Involuntary spasms of your pelvic muscles are undoubtedly one of the most pleasurable parts of coming. Flexing your sexual muscles intentionally is another powerful way you can use the movement cornerstone to generate, spread, and circulate orgasmic energy.

We're referring to your *pubococcygeal* muscles located at your pelvic floor.

As figure 11 on page 92 shows, the layers of pelvic muscles are shaped like a figure eight that surrounds and supports the jewels in both men and women. To identify them, put one of your hands on your pubic bone. That's the one above your jewels, below your tummy, and under your pubic hair.

Now reach around and put your other hand near the top of your butt crack at the very bottom of your spine. The pelvic floor muscles connect these bones, plus your sitting bones and legs. They snake down around your jewels and rosetta.

It's more important to identify these muscles from the inside. They're the ones you hold when you don't want to pee.

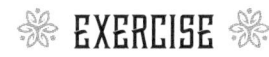

EXERCISE
Find Your Pelvic Floor Muscles

1. Try squeezing your pelvic floor muscles right now. Did you feel them?
2. If not, go to the toilet. Start peeing and stop in the middle.
3. When you're finished, try to squeeze the last few drops out. The muscles you used to stop and squeeze are the ones we're referring to.

Pelvic Floor Benefits

Having strong pelvic muscles, keeping them relaxed, and using them without strain can dramatically enhance your sexual pleasure. Why?

First off, your sexual muscles pulse rhythmically during orgasm, releasing tension, fluids, and sexual energy. If they're weak, your contractions will be, too. If they're strong, you can use them to consciously pump the energy out of your jewels and spread the pleasure up your inner flute.

The yoni of a woman with well-toned pelvic floor muscles will be healthier and produce stronger sensations. And she can use the ancient Asian and Arabian art of *pompoir* to grasp, grip, and massage a visiting vajra.

A man's erections and ability to regulate premature ejaculation also depend on strong sexual muscles. The payoff for men with toned sexual muscles includes longer stamina, stronger orgasms, and prostate health.

Chronic tension in the pelvic floor blocks the flow of energy up and down the inner flute. Exercising these muscles will help you overcome the natural tendency to tighten up during sexual arousal. If your muscles are well toned, you can consciously relax them and stream sexual energy more easily.

Consequently, we suggest you start a regimen of daily sexual muscle exercises. They're similar to the post-childbirth exercises developed by the gynecologist Dr. Arnold Kegel in 1952. Most people call these internal squeezes *Kegels*.[8]

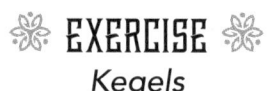

EXERCISE
Kegels

1. To strengthen your pelvic floor muscles, all you have to do is squeeze and hold them for a few seconds as though you were trying to stop urinating midstream. After each contraction, relax for the same amount of time.
2. Pump your muscles a dozen times during your first set.
3. Then add one or two more sets daily.
4. Gradually increase, holding the contractions for up to one minute and the number of reps in each of the three sets up to thirty. Initially expect it will take you several weeks to get where you want to be.
5. Find a time and place where you'll remember to do your Kegels. You might use reminders like when you stop for traffic lights, check your email, see a TV commercial, or start your workout at the gym.

5. Visualization

Visualization, which simply means to picture something in your mind's eye, is the last cornerstone of ecstasy. At a sexual peak, your mind can't help but be consumed with pleasure. Put your most powerful sex organ, your mind, consciously to work. Use what naturally happens as an intentional tool.

---

8. Margot Anand, *The Art of Sexual Ecstasy* (Los Angeles: Tarcher, 1989), 175–179.

The power of visualization stems from the principle that states that "energy flows where attention goes."⁹ Create a mental image of the sensations you want. Put your attention where you want more pleasure to flow.

When you focus your attention on any body part you want to heat up, you attract lifeforce there. When you imagine sexual juice and electricity building in a sweet spot, you attract erotic charge there.

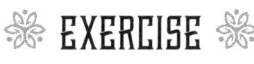

EXERCISE
Visualization

1. To practice visualization, sit comfortably and focus on your breath.
2. Start by picturing energy moving in your body.
3. Now visualize there's a red-hot fire in front of you. Imagine drawing in a golden ball of radiant light from the fire through your first chakra with your in-breath. Feel the warmth seeping into your loins.
4. Watch the energy stream back to the fire on the out-breath.
5. Next, visualize pulling the pictured energy up your inner flute to your heart on the next in-breath. Try it for a few minutes to see how it makes you feel.

This was one of the first Tantric exercises we regularly practiced to meld the energies of sex and love. Later we did the same at each chakra, ultimately connecting our jewels and hearts with the Divine. Because this cornerstone depends on quieting the mind, the power of visualization greatly depends on the first cornerstone: presence.

Putting It Together with Orgasmic Breathing

You can use each of the five cornerstones of ecstasy for specific purposes at different times. Presence helps you relax and be more conscious. The Tantric breath spreads your kundalini and making love sounds amplifies it. Pelvic rocking frees your channels and Kegels shoot energy up your inner flute. Visualization directs your kundalini where you want it to flow.

---

9. https://www.goodreads.com/quotes/816367-where-attention-goes-energy-flows-where-intention-goes-energy-flows.

Synchronizing all five cornerstones is the most powerful. We call that the learned skill of *orgasmic breathing*. To breathe orgasmically, clear your mind, get totally absorbed in your feelings, breathe deeper through your mouth (the Tantric breath), let your love sounds loose, erotically gyrate your bodies, pump your pelvic muscles, and visualize kundalini streaming.

Orgasmic breathing is the way you expand your pleasure balloon to fill your biofield. Then you can circulate the sexual forces to your higher chakras instead of releasing all that delicious energy too soon. When you want to reach a higher peak or relax in an orgasmic plateau, your visualizations have much more power. It's also the key to exchanging kundalini at multiple levels.

Orgasmic breathing is doing what your body already knows how to do while climaxing. But when you do it willfully, your pleasure builds. If you've practiced each of the five cornerstones, all you must do is coordinate the separate parts.

❊ EXERCISE ❊
Orgasmic Breathing

1. Practice orgasmic breathing by yourself at first to get all the pieces to fit comfortably and naturally. Before you begin, play some slow, sensuous music. Sit and breathe until you're feeling present in the here and now.
2. When you're relaxed, add pelvic rocking. You can rotate your hips forward on your in-breath and back on your out-breath. Or the opposite if it feels more natural.
3. When you're ready, squeeze your pelvic floor muscles on your in-breath. Release them on your out-breath.
4. Next, start making love sounds on your out-breaths.
5. When you're in a groove with the previous pieces, add the final step, visualization. Imagine energy coming into your first chakra on your in-breath and being pumped up to your heart by your Kegels. Follow it streaming out your pelvis on the out-breath.
6. In later practice sessions, visualize the energy moving up to the other chakras, eventually all the way to the crown of the head.

7. Next, try it with your partner. Sit across from each other with your eyes closed. Separately do orgasmic breathing until you've settled into a routine. Then open your eyes and synchronize your breathing.

Orgasmic breathing can propel any kind of lovemaking to reach spectacular heights of sexual ecstasy.[10]

Summary and Action Steps

- Consciously use the five cornerstones to amplify your ecstasy.
- Develop the presence cornerstone by staying in the moment, feeling your body, releasing your thoughts, and clearing your mind.
- Practice breathing Tantrically with the Tantric Breath Exercise.
- Make a genuine effort to vocalize love sounds. Open your throat (fifth chakra) with the Love Sounds Exercise.
- Do yoga or pelvic stretching to loosen up your body.
- Amplify your turn-on with the Erotic Movement Exercise.
- Create a daily regimen of Kegel exercises.
- Learn to move energy with the Visualization Exercise.
- Practice the Orgasmic Breathing Exercise and then incorporate it into your lovemaking.

---

10. Margot Anand, *The Art of Sexual Ecstasy* (Los Angeles: Tarcher, 1989), 179–183.

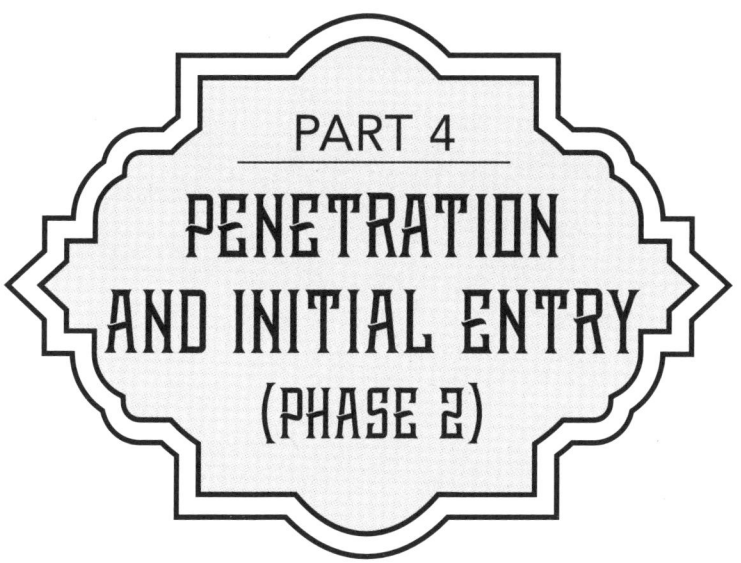

PART 4
PENETRATION AND INITIAL ENTRY
(PHASE 2)

At last we will directly address jewel union. PART 4 relates the first steps in penetrating a yoni or a rosetta. Here you'll read about initial entry, sex positions, rosetta (anal) sex, and energetic *armoring*. The latter is what we call a body's tendency to store tension and resistance from past traumas.

Even though much of this applies to same-sex lovemaking, we hope you don't mind us using "he" and "she" to simplify things.

Supernatural Sex is a joy for all kinds of partnered lovers. We strive to include all sexual preferences in our explanations. Hopefully you'll see that everything fully applies to you in spite of these language limitations.

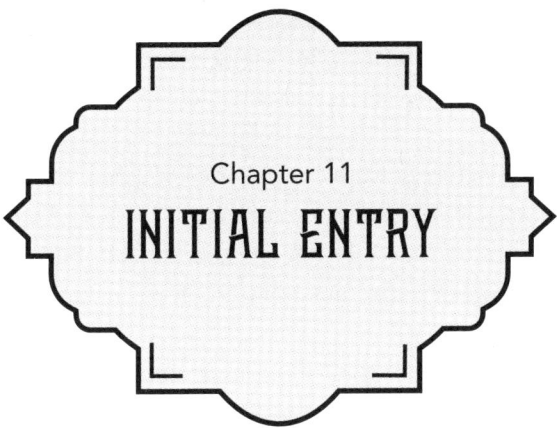

Chapter 11
INITIAL ENTRY

A woman's yoni must be fully awakened before she can really enjoy jewel union. We urge you to make sure your partner's yoni is fully erect and engorged before receiving a vajra. Even when she's craving penetration, just shoving it in and going to town isn't recommended.

The purpose of this chapter is to make sure that penetration begins erotically instead of traumatically, that it establishes and maintains a sweet, loving energy connection, and that it prevents premature penetration and ejaculation.

Initial Entry

Initial entry is when a man's vajra first penetrates a yoni or rosetta. Let's start with the yoni, an amazingly elastic cavity that is potentially highly supple and responsive. This expandable complex of muscles and tissues can pass a baby's head with proper preparation.

But yonis don't open instantly. Even the most active yonis need time to relax, warm up, and stretch around an entering vajra.

When a yoni is assaulted too suddenly by waves of overwhelming sensation, it can constrict uncomfortably or even painfully. If a woman is inexperienced, out of practice, anxious, or overly cautious, this adjustment can take many minutes. If she has a medical condition affecting her jewels or has been the victim of sexual abuse or violence, her yoni may be unnaturally tense or completely blocked.

Extensive loveplay creating a full female erection gives a woman's body ample time to adjust through lots of easy, low-pressure titillation. That's when initial entry can begin with slow, gentle, and sensitive movements. Sometimes that means holding still until she relaxes and welcomes a vajra inside. Ideally you will both wait until his vajra is virtually pulled inside instead of forcing its way in.

In this delicate juncture, a vajra can provide a much-needed service of helping a woman's yoni release tension, awaken to pleasure, and open to kundalini flows. You make contact delicately and lovingly until she becomes accustomed to what's penetrating her. Hurrying and using force reduces her comfort and may trigger old baggage.

Sure, there are occasions when the primal animal needs and wants to be ravished by a savage beast. If you get such clear signals, you can dispense with the initial measured caution we suggest. We just don't recommend it without familiarity. If it's your first time together, asking how she wants it is a great addition to the partnering questions. Even if you've made love before, there's no guarantee that what thrilled her then will do so now.

It's difficult for many men to truly appreciate how shocking vigorous initial entry can be. The first time Somraj's rosetta was penetrated gave him a new level of appreciation of the supreme sensitivity that's needed. Now he slides into a yoni deliberately instead of plunging in wildly. As well, slow insertion thrusts help a man settle into the extreme initial jolt of sensation and avoid premature ejaculation.

Initial entry is best in a safe, loving atmosphere. The Tantric attitude is essential. Take your time and savor every little bit of pleasure. You both want to be fully present and totally conscious to experience the intense sensations of jewel union.

This measured approach to initial entry is the responsibility of both partners. We suggest the following

1. Communicate before you dominate.
2. Monitor each other's reactions.
3. Take your time until you find a comfortable groove and a sweet rhythm that pleases you both.

Initial Entry Cues

Ancient sex manuals devoted a lot of attention to knowing when a woman is ready be entered. We call these *initial entry cues*.

Initial entry cues include her face flushing, her ears getting hot and turning red, her nostrils flaring, her breasts swelling, and goose bumps spreading everywhere. The time may be right if she opens her mouth, breathes deeper, and moans with desire. You'll know what to do if she reaches for you, spreads her legs, and rubs her privates against yours.

Valuable advice, no doubt, but it's more reliable to pay attention to the state of her yoni's erection. Better yet, ask if she's ready. Or wait until she requests, demands, or even begs for penetration.

The popular myth that men are always ready for sex doesn't work for Supernatural Sex. A quick hard-on doesn't guarantee that a guy's energy channels are open and firing. Somraj is often put off when his vajra is fondled before the rest of his body is excited. Otherwise he has trouble raising the energy up from his jewels to enjoy all-chakra lovemaking.

Are he and his vajra energetically primed for entry? Instead of blindly assuming if a guy is hard he's ready, we suggest you check first. If his erection is a bit soft, you might try a *hand-assist*. That means using fingers to guide his vajra toward and into yoni's mouth. An empowered lover can grab, fondle, or suck him for a bit. Or he can stroke his vajra with his hand. He could also massage his vajra's head on her erect yoni.

On the other hand, he might be too sensitive to dive inside right now. This isn't the time to put pressure on him to perform. Avoiding premature ejaculation is a joint responsibility for enlightened lovers.

One option is loveplay until his excitement settles down. He could bring his partner to orgasm with his mouth before penetration to offset the orgasm gap.

A sensual massage elsewhere on his body may help him spread the energy away from his nearly spasming love tool. She could help him reach several pleasure peaks with her hand or mouth without going over the top. This lessens the sensitivity of most men. Or maybe she could get him off if he can recover quickly with less sensitivity.

In short, check in with each other as needed instead of expecting the actors will always perform perfectly.

✻ EXERCISE ✻
Initial Entry Discussion

1. Read the previous sections together.
2. Talk about earlier times when initial entry has been pleasurable.
3. Talk about earlier times when it wasn't.
4. Discuss what you want to do in the future.

First Contact

That first contact between vajra's head and yoni's lips can be scary and shocking, or erotic and electric, or both. Handling it tenderly and consciously is crucial.

Remember, Supernatural Sex is a team effort. Sometimes he'll take charge. That's when asking permission with something like "Are you ready to be entered?" is a nice touch. This is when you put on a condom or apply some lube, if necessary.

The woman can also take charge of first contact. Whoever is leading, hold vajra's head or shaft against her moist, puffy lips. Don't move much at first. Using orgasmic breathing will help you both relax and focus on the sensations.

One of our favorite ways to insure we're both ready for initial entry is with a *vajra yoni-massage*. You do this by one of you rubbing outer yoni using a hand-assist, particularly yoni's mouth, with vajra's head.

You don't need an erection to play with vajra yoni-massage. This can be even more delightful with a soft member. And it's highly effective in turning a soft stalk into a hard pole.

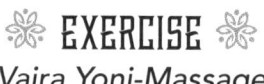
EXERCISE
Vajra Yoni-Massage

1. Rest vajra's head against your partner's yoni. Then slide the shaft between yoni's lips.
2. Either of you can grab his organ and rub it up and down and around outer yoni.
3. Play around this way from her mound, across her vestibule, and down to her perineum. Be sure to churn around yoni's mouth and outlet.
4. When she's ready, massage her clio with vajra's head.

That First Inch

We know the first contact of your jewels might make that voice in your head scream to shove it all the way. Please don't. Instead, take a deep breath and pause before penetration.

When her body is asking for more, either of you can lovingly spread her lips with your fingers. Then insert vajra's first inch inside her puffy cuff. Take your time and let vajra's head caress the first inch inside of yoni's mouth until she relaxes.

Let her yoni's loosening tell you when she's ready for more. Neither of you want to force his vajra past that first band of muscles protecting her yoni's opening.

Focus on the touch of each other's wet, hot, or hard engorged tissues. Put all your attention on feeling the delightful sensations sparking between your jewels. Do you feel the vibrations, the contractions, the electricity? What else is happening in your body, your heart, your mind? Savor whatever the feelings are. If you like, share what you're both experiencing.

Repeat

Then, slowly pull out a bit—not all the way—and pause for a few seconds. You want to maintain the electrical and energetic connection during this critical process.

Repeat the glacially slow one-inch thrust a few times if she's responding passionately. Let vajra's head descend slowly, softly, and sensitively each time without rushing, pushing, or forcing. Your aim during these first measured strokes is to feel more than pump.

You're waiting until you feel a softening, a relaxing, a welcoming, almost as if yoni is sucking vajra deeper. Only then do you gingerly try another inch and repeat the whole measured process.

Though this is a team effort, it's important for the man to hold back his wild animal. Let her know she shares the decision power. Make this a sacred ritual that honors her. It's more about building trust and awakening kundalini than making her come right away. In fact, an empowered woman can take the lead.

Deeper

Continue your first thrusts a little deeper when her reaction is positive. Test if she's ready for a little faster, too. You can gradually build depth and speed if you find her body is clearly enjoying it.

How many slow, shallow thrusts does it take? The glib answer is it takes as long as it takes. Let her yoni decide. If you pay close attention, you'll know when she's ready for faster, harder, and deeper. Only when her cuff is inflamed and her body is asking for more is it time to move deeper. Or you can ask.

Maybe you need just one or two first thrusts before the action heats up. Or maybe one long, slow thrust all the way to the hilt is what she's craving. Or maybe she'll enjoy a few minutes of gradually going deeper and speeding up. Just don't make these early strokes too vigorous too soon.

How fast you can enter into fast pumping depends on many factors, including how fast her yoni awakens and your relative jewel size. If his girth stretches her yoni too much, take longer. If she's looser inside, you might be able to proceed more swiftly.

Sometimes everything feels great for the first few inches, but then you hit a wall. It's most likely a tender or armored spot. If that happens, back off and proceed even more gradually.

All the Way

As you go deeper, try shifting your angle of entry up or down or side to side. Maybe she'll adore you circling your hips to probe all of yoni's inner walls in the same tender manner.

But we haven't arrived at full uninhibited jewel union yet. The emphasis here is still on opening her yoni. It's up to the two of you to decide when the time is right to go all the way.

It's her job to let him know if she wants it faster or slower, deeper or shallower, harder or softer. And to naturally and uninhibitedly show her turn-ons. His job is to watch her reactions, read her cues, and ask how things feel. Is her yoni expanding, heating up, and getting more receptive?

Sometimes this excruciatingly slow process we've described might be more cautious than is actually necessary. But we wanted to make sure you know how to be the most tender lover in recorded history. By the way, you may want to return to this initial entry regimen after a break, if you hit a snag, to add a little teasing, or simply to add variety.

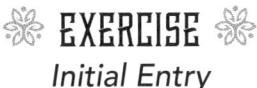
Initial Entry

1. Read this chapter together and then discuss the partnering questions.
2. Enjoy some loveplay until you're both ready for penetration.
3. Begin with some vajra yoni-massage.
4. Then, by agreement, one of you slowly inserts the vajra the first inch a few times.
5. When you're ready, stroke a bit at a depth of two inches.
6. Go deeper when the time is right.

Soft Entry

A flagging erection can be a major impediment to Supernatural Sex, especially as men age or encounter medical issues. *Soft entry* is a workable solution that removes the pressure to always be hard.

It is possible to insert a soft love tool by offering a helping hand, literally. Here's how Tantra teacher Diana Richardson explains a special form of hand-assist in her great book *The Heart of Tantric Sex*.[11] It's relatively easy for either partner once you develop the knack of soft entry.

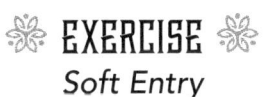
Soft Entry

1. Get into a sexual position that brings your pelvises close together. Missionary works, but our favorite is the Scissors Position where we lie down at right angles to each other and intertwine our legs.
2. One of you holds his vajra with a two-pronged fork using the first two fingers of one hand. Apply some lubricant, but not enough so his vajra is too slippery.
3. Firmly hold the base of his vajra with one finger-fork and grip his vajra just below the crown with a finger-fork on the other hand. Squeeze just

---

11. Diana Richardson, *The Heart of Tantric Sex* (Alresford, UK: O Books, 2003), 116–118.

enough to maintain control and pull his vajra toward her yoni. With an uncircumcised organ, pull back the foreskin to expose vajra's head.

4. As your jewels meet, push vajra's head inside yoni's mouth, keeping a firm grip with the base finger-fork. Then slide the crown finger-fork down a bit and push in again.
5. Repeat this maneuver a few times to feed his vajra inside bit by bit. When his vajra is as deep as it can go, remove your hands, bring your pelvises closely together, and relax.

You may not feel much at first. But gradually you should feel a subtle tingling or a faint electrical buzzing. The innate magnetic polarity gradually creates a sexual energy flow between your jewels. Given a little time, they awaken and do their thing as nature intended. Then all you have to do is enjoy it.

If you haven't made love for some time, rarely enjoyed it, or have had some painful sexual traumas, your jewels may be somewhat desensitized. It takes some faith in the technique to benefit from and enjoy soft entry. Approach this process with as few expectations as possible. With any luck, his stalk will grow hard enough for stroking. If not, it's still a fun way to create some good feelings.

Summary and Action Steps

- Take your time and prevent premature penetration.
- Do the Initial Entry Discussion Exercise to decide how you want to handle it in the future.
- Ask permission before penetration.
- Look for cues that you're both ready.
- Begin initial entry slowly, gently, and sensitively.
- Use vajra yoni-massage for first contact.
- Carefully stroke one inch deep at first. Then try two inches.
- Only let your thrusting get deeper and harder when she and her yoni ask for it.
- Use the Soft Entry Exercise when you need it.

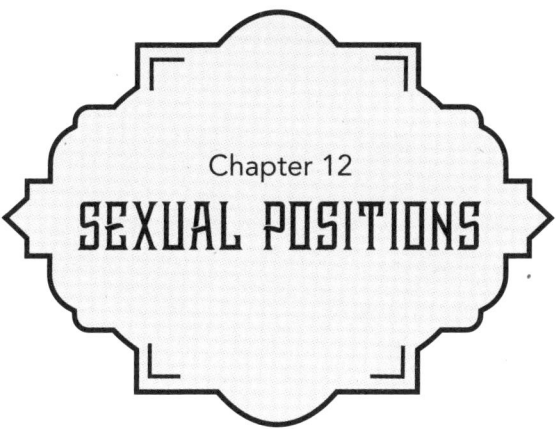

Chapter 12
SEXUAL POSITIONS

When you extend jewel union past a quick draining explosion, you open the door to enjoying multiple sexual positions. Every human body is different. When your two different bodies couple, how you connect is unique. Some positions feel better than others. Some are kinky and exciting, some channel more kundalini, and some strain certain types of bodies. No matter how much fun you're having, you'll probably get tired of most positions after a while.

Variety is an essential element of maximizing sexual energy in Supernatural Sex. Plus, morphing in and out of postures helps you search for sweet spots and more. In this chapter we'll review the full spectrum of sexual positions available to you and how to shift to create more pleasure.

Jewel Sizes

The *Kama Sutra* and other treatises from India and China are well known for their graphic description of sexual positions. Curiously, their recommendations were based on relative jewel sizes of men and women. What's not clear is how lovers discovered the dimensions of a potential mate's private-parts.

Regardless, when you begin jewel union you'll quickly learn how it's working. Part of the *Kama Sutra's* appeal is describing how to compensate for maximum comfort and pleasure.

Basically, big yonis are happier with big vajras. Mediums prefer mediums, and small ones love small ones. But if you heed this ancient wisdom, you can compensate whatever your relative dimensions and have lots of fun.

Ancient erotic manuals classified yonis based on depth: [12]

Deer	Five inches deep
Mare	Seven inches deep
Elephant	Ten inches deep

Vajras were classified based on length when fully erect:

Hare	Five inches long
Bull	Seven inches long
Stallion	Ten inches long

Modern surveys have shown the average erect penis is between five and six inches long. Some are thicker, some are thinner, some are harder, and some are fleshier.[13]

The average unexcited yoni is around three inches deep unstimulated, ample enough for the overwhelming majority of vajras in the world.[14] So, though these traditional ratings seem larger than today's norms, the whole concept of matching relative sizes still holds.

Equal and Unequal Relations

The *Kama Sutra* called the best match with same-sized jewels *equal relations*. That includes small with small, medium with medium, and large with large.

With equal relations, penetration is easy. The woman doesn't need to open or contract her yoni. The man need not aspire to athletic postures for a tighter or more comfortable fit.

Unequal relations are between lovers with different-sized jewels. There are different levels of unequal relations, the more unequal the more difficult for comfort and satisfaction.

Highest Union	Largest vajra with smallest yoni
High Union	Vajra one size larger than the yoni

---

12. Wendy Doniger and Sudhir Kakar, *Kamasutra* (New York: Oxford University Press, 2002), 28.
13. David Veale et. al, "Am I Normal?," Wiley.com, December 8, 2014, https://onlinelibrary.wiley.com/doi/full/10.1111/bju.13010.
14. TammyWorth, "Does Vagina Size Matter?" WebMD.com, July 20, 2011, https://www.webmd.com/women/features/vagina-size#1.

Low Union	Yoni one size larger than vajra
Lowest Union	Smallest vajra with largest yoni

You know that yonis can expand, as demonstrated by the tremendous expansion during birth. Thus, the potential exists to accommodate highest unions with pleasure instead of pain.

If you're a deer woman (smallest) or stallion man (largest), you've likely been in this situation. Rushing into a quickie probably won't work. You'll need extra loveplay, a fully erect yoni cuff, and slower first thrusts.

In high and highest unions, you want to choose sexual positions that allow the woman to open and stretch her yoni. If she spreads her thighs, she'll make yoni's inside space bigger for vajras with bigger girth. Bigger space also accommodates longer members more easily and allows them deeper access. Still, stallion men need to be cautious about how far they penetrate.

Both men and women can compensate for low and lowest unions. Ancient texts advise that a woman with a larger yoni uses her muscles and sex positions to tighten her canal. Regular pelvic floor exercises are vital.

Isn't it fascinating there's so much attention on vajra size today and so little on yoni strength and suppleness? Other cultures encouraged women to master pompoir, the yoni skill of gripping and milking inserted male members that we introduced in chapter 10 about the five cornerstones of ecstasy.

The discipline of cautious first thrusts isn't as vital with low and lowest unions as it is in other cases. But if you're worried that your coupling isn't tight enough, consider this: How large is the opening of the average yoni? Zero. Yes, at rest, yoni walls press against each other.

So just about any vajra can make adequate contact with enough of a yoni to create the seeds of great pleasure.

Sexual Positions and Postures

Some sexual positions are easy, and some are challenging. Some work for mature bodies and others don't. And some are better for same-sex lovers than others.

Within each sexual position there are various ways you can shift your bodies. Create these sexual *postures* by moving your torsos, adjusting your limbs, and shifting your weight. Here's how we define sexual positions and the primary postures of each, along with an illustration of one posture.

Man-Above Position

(Missionary: she's on her back, he's on top.)

> Her Legs Close: he's between her legs as she squeezes hers close.
> Her Legs Wide: her thighs are wide, he's between her legs.
> He Rolls Upward: he moves toward her chest with her legs together or wide.
> Her Legs Up: her legs are high.
> Holding: she holds his waist tight with her legs.
> Flanquette: he's at an angle over her.
> Surrounding: his legs are on either side of hers, which are together.

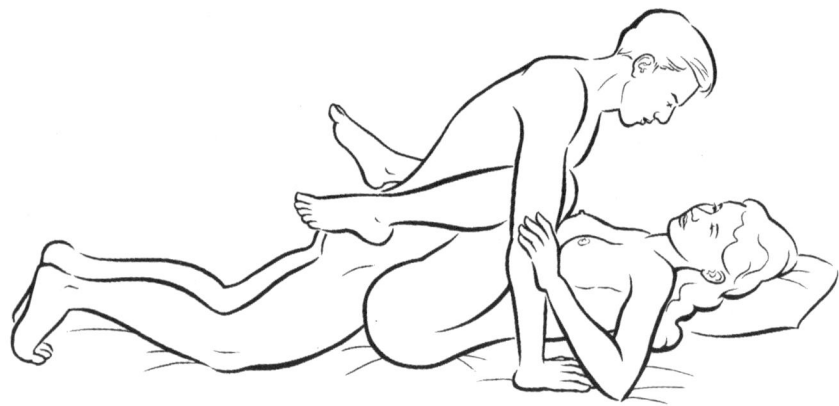

Figure 12: Man-Above Position, Her Legs Up Posture

Man-Kneeling Position

(She's on her back, he kneels between her legs.)

Wide Open: her body is raised up with legs wide.

Holding: she holds his waist tight with her legs.

Chest: her feet or knees are on his chest.

Shoulders: her feet are on his shoulders.

Head: her feet are on his head.

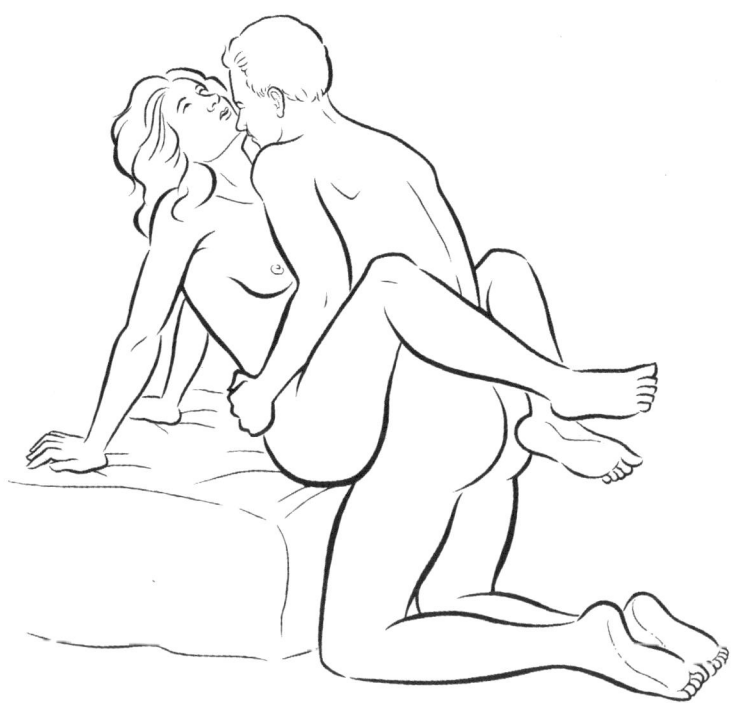

Figure 13: Man-Kneeling Position, Holding Posture

Woman-Above Position

(Cowgirl: she's on top, he's on his back.)

> Kneeling Forward: she kneels over, facing his head.
>
> Squatting Forward: she squats over, facing his head.
>
> Lying Forward: she lies forward on top of him.
>
> Sitting on Top: she sits on top of him.
>
> Facing Backward: she sits, squats, kneels, or lies facing his feet (Reverse Cowgirl).

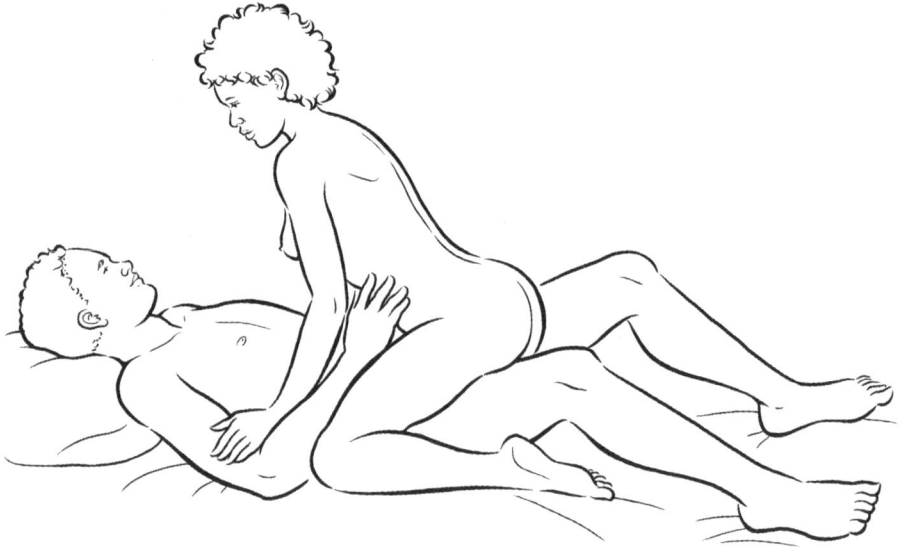

Figure 14: Woman-Above Position, Kneeling Forward Posture

Rear-Entry Position

(Doggie Style: she's on all fours, he's behind her.)

> Doggie: she's on all fours with him behind.
>
> Bent Over: she's on her knees with her shoulders on the bed, he's behind.
>
> Facedown: she lies facedown with legs wide, he's on top.
>
> Surrounding: she's facedown with legs together, he's on top with legs outside hers.
>
> Spoon: she's on her side, he lies behind her on his side.

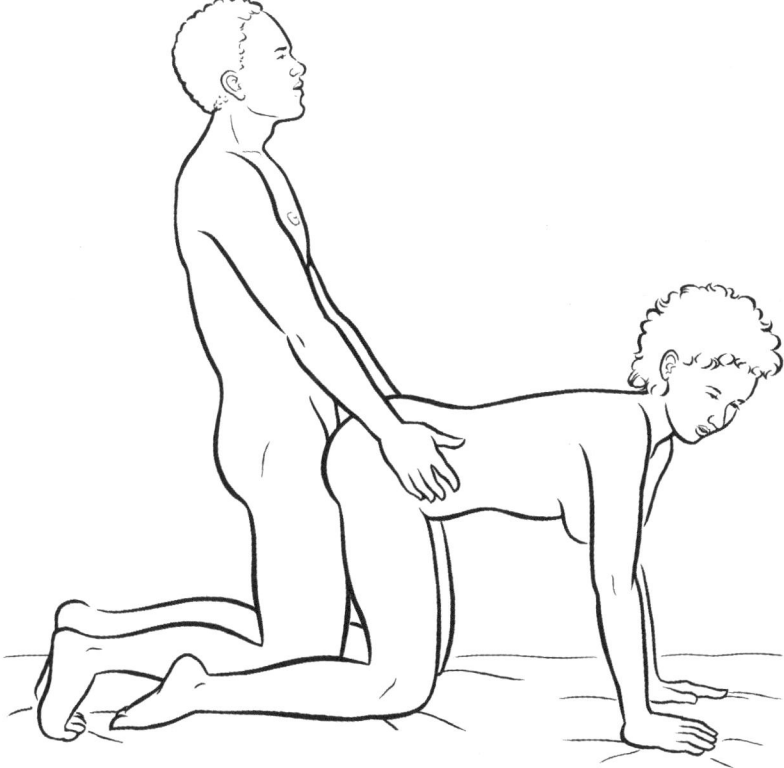

Figure 15: Rear-Entry Position, Doggie Style Posture

Side-to-Side Position

(Both are lying down.)

Woman on Back: she's on her back, he's at right angles with legs under hers.

Scissors: similar to Woman on Back but with legs intertwined.

Woman on Side: she's on her side, he kneels behind her.

Facing: they face each other, both on their sides.

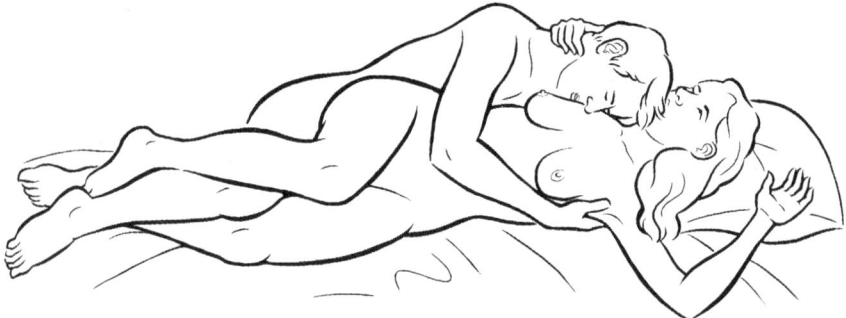

Figure 16: Side-to-Side Position

Sitting Position
(Both are sitting with legs arranged creatively.)

Yab-Yum: he sits cross-legged with her on his lap facing him.

Straddling: they straddle one another with one or more legs.

Raised: he sits cross-legged, she's on his lap with her legs raised.

Leaning: leaning back partway or all the way from Yab-Yum.

Reverse: he sits cross-legged with her on his lap facing away from him.

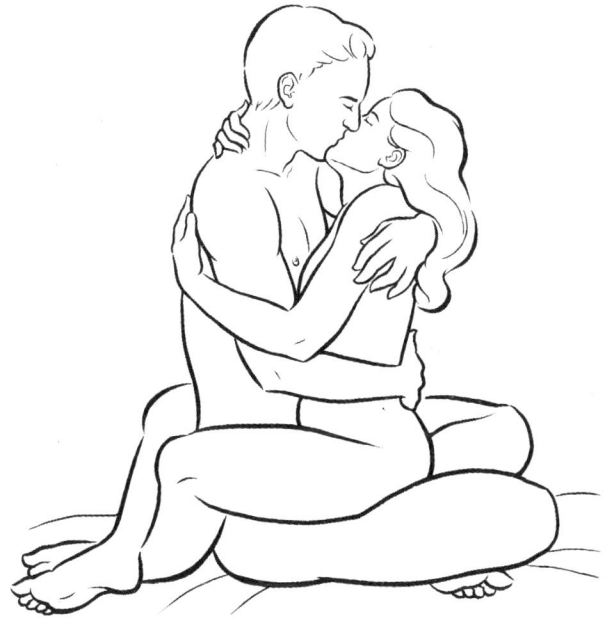

Figure 17: Sitting Position, Yab-Yum Posture

Chapter 12

Standing Position
(Both are standing up, usually with some kind of support.)

Facing: both stand facing each other.
Reverse: she leans against a wall or couch, he stands behind her.
Suspended: he holds her up so she's suspended from his body.
Bed or Table: she lies on her back, he stands between her legs.
Love Swing: she lies in a hammock, he stands between her legs.

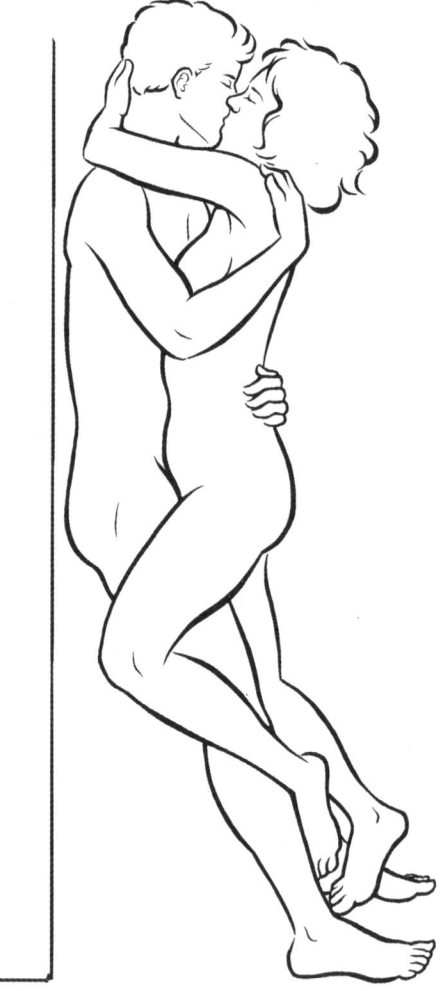

Figure 18: Standing Position, Facing Posture

Choosing Postures

Because some body arrangements hit certain sweet spots and some don't, different lovers have their favorite postures. You have to balance excitement against comfort. Many sexual postures derive from yoga asanas (poses). If you don't practice yoga, many of them may be too physically demanding. No matter, you still have an ample variety of exciting alternatives.

One of Jeffre's hips gets tired pretty quickly, so we rarely spend much time in a Side-to-Side Position that puts all her weight on her right side. Somraj loves giving Rear-Entry penetration, but it's not the easiest for us to maintain. Besides, it just doesn't hit many sweet spots inside Jeffre's yoni. We both love the Man-Above surrounding posture for its tight fit and intense clio stimulation. But with some lovers it can quickly rub yoni's lips raw.

Relative body size is a primary factor in finding comfortable ways to enjoy jewel union. A much smaller lover will probably be happier on top. Your strength and flexibility figure in, as do any physical limitations that either of you have. For example, our lower backs can get out of whack if we hold a strained position for too long.

Standing Positions are popular in porn, but only very strong lovers can hold them easily for long. Even in the Man-Above Position, our arms can only prop us up for so long before getting tired and aching.

Comfort isn't just a nicety. Any part of your body that's under strain can block the flow of kundalini. If an arm, leg, back, or butt gets numb or painful while making love, don't ignore it. Speak up and shift as soon as you can.

Selecting postures that allow for the most pleasurable stroking is a joint responsibility based on how your unique bodies fit. How tight is your particular vajra in her one-of-a-kind yoni? How deep does your vajra go? Does her clio get stimulated at all? Does your vajra hit her G-crest?

These kinds of considerations determine how turned-on you both get, how quickly you approach orgasm, and how long you can last.

Other Considerations

Some postures allow you to fondle your own or your partner's jewels or add a vibrator to the mix. Other poses naturally define who's dominating and who's submitting.

Watching the in-and-out action is often a huge turn-on. It's easier for men than women in many postures. Postures in the Man-Kneeling or Woman-Above Positions afford her a free erotic show. Mirrors on the wall or ceiling and hand mirrors can add a spicy addition.

There are many ways to connect other chakras during jewel union. Eye contact, kissing, caressing, sharing sweet everythings, and other forms of communicating are easier when you're face-to-face. This encourages a closer heart, stronger energy, and unified spiritual connection. Aligning your chakras next to each other makes it easier to exchange and circulate kundalini. The Man-Above and Sitting Positions facilitate these kinds of intimacy, but Rear-Entry Positions don't.

We encourage you to try the whole range of lovemaking positions and find what makes your sex supernatural.

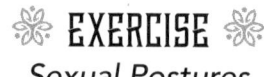

EXERCISE
Sexual Postures

1. Read this chapter together.
2. Decide if your jewels unite in an equal, low, or high union.
3. Review the sexual positions and postures and decide what you'd like to experiment with.
4. Enjoy some jewel union and try out what you've planned.
5. Afterward, talk about how it worked and what you'd like to try next time.

Hitting Sweet Spots

The most important consideration in choosing sexual positions is how well a posture lets your jewels hit each other's sweet spots. We encourage you to freely experiment and communicate during jewel union. You can adjust vajra's depth and angle of entry by shifting your bodies or using pillows.

In many postures of the Man-Above and Man-Kneeling Positions, vajra's head enters from above. Various postures of the Woman-Above Position, the Standing Position, and the facing posture of the Side-to-Side Position do the same. Elevating his pelvis or lowering hers by putting her legs down or raising her body with pillows increases this angle.

Shallow strokes in these postures cause vajra's head to strike the woman's lower sponge around yoni's bottom wall. Thrusts that are a little deeper slide vajra's shaft firmly against her G-crest while vajra's head pummels her lower sponge.

On the other hand, when a vajra enters shallowly from a low angle, the shaft rubs a woman's lower sponge and the head impacts her G-crest directly. Low, shallow entry is the natural consequence of the Side-to-Side and Sitting Positions and most postures of the Rear-Entry Position. The woman can accentuate low entry in positions like Man-Above by raising her legs and rotating her pelvis up.

Somewhat deeper thrusts that enter from high, middle, or low may prod the plexi on either side of yoni's canal when they enter from left or right.

Relative body size also affects how a vajra enters a yoni in all postures. In the Rear-Entry or Standing Positions, a man with shorter legs will hit the G-crest and rub the lower sponge of a longer-legged woman. If his pelvis is higher, he'll hit the lower sponge and rub her G-crest.

Deep Yoni Stimulation

Many women enjoy cervix and fornix (the A-spot and cul-de-sac) stimulation. Though some find this uncomfortable, it can possibly be corrected with yoni clearing, which we'll address later.

Prodding these sweet spots requires deep penetration, which can be accomplished in a wide variety of sexual positions such as the Man-Above with Her Legs Up, Man-Kneeling with her legs wide, Woman-Above with Sitting on Top, Rear-Entry on all fours, and Reverse Standing.

Straight insertion in these positions targets the cervix directly. High, deep entry, as in the above positions, stimulates the cul-de-sac. Low, deep entry jostles the A-spot. The more extreme vajra's upward angle, the more he can target her A-spot toward her stomach. In the most extreme angle, he can stroke along her engorged urethral sponge behind her pubic bone.

If the length of your vajra doesn't hit these deep sweet spots, you may want to experiment with a dildo or sex toy called a *penis extender*.

Targeting Clio

When a vajra enters a yoni, it stretches the inner lips inward. Since the lips are attached to clio's hood, to some degree the pulling stimulates clio's pearl and shaft. All sorts of sexual strokes massage the V-bulbs and clio's crura when yoni is erect. Tight yoni positions like postures with her legs together and surrounding postures increase both kinds of erotic friction.

Studies show that 70 percent of women need clio stimulation to orgasm during jewel union.[15] Unfortunately, the pearl of only 10 percent of women is close enough to yoni's mouth to receive direct stimulation from vajra's shaft during normal thrusting.[16] The rest need something more.

Penetrating from a very steep angle from above such as in the Man-Above Position with him rolling upward stimulates the woman's outlet and clio's pearl. In this posture he can swipe clio's pearl and shaft as his vajra enters and withdraws.

Because clio's shaft rests on top of the pubic bone, another way to impact clio during jewel union is with *pubic grinding*. This is when a man rubs and grinds his pubic bone against the woman's in various postures of Man-Above or Man-Kneeling Positions. A woman on top can rotate her clio down as his vajra enters and roll upward firmly against his shaft.

With his vajra all the way inside, you can linger there, press firmly, and grind. The one above can rock side to side, slide up and down, or rotate the pubic bone in circles over her clio.

We'll address stimulating clio by hand or vibrator later.

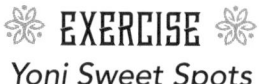

Yoni Sweet Spots

1. Read the previous sections together.
2. Discuss how jewel union could better contact yoni and clio's sweet spots.
3. Test out your plans during jewel union.

---

15. Lizette Borelli. "The Sex Moves Women Want: Clitoral Stimulation Helps Female Orgasm, Study Finds." Newsweek.com. 9/21/2017. https://www.newsweek.com/sex-moves-female-orgasm-relationships-dating-669154.

16. Ally Hirschlag. "Why Some Women Orgasm Easier Than Others." SheKnows.com. 5/6/2016. https://www.sheknows.com/love-and-sex/articles/1120927/why-some-women-have-better-orgasms.

The above examples are only a few of the ways you can contact a woman's sweet spots during jewel union. There is much more to learn by experimenting. As you play, also consider how you're arousing the man's erogenous zones.

Summary and Action Steps

- When you choose a lover, consider relative jewel sizes.
- If your jewel fit is tight or loose, learn to compensate with creative sex positions.
- Choose sexual postures that are both comfortable and exciting.
- Do the Sexual Postures Exercise together if you have a current lover.
- Speak up and shift if any part of your body gets numb or sore.
- Freely experiment and communicate during jewel union to find which sexual postures best hit your sweet spots.
- Stimulate her clio during jewel union with pubic grinding.
- Do the Yoni Sweet Spots Exercise to learn more about what she likes.

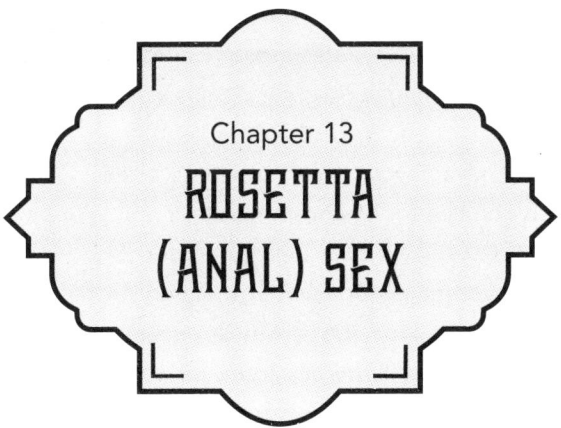

Chapter 13
ROSETTA (ANAL) SEX

The yoni is not the only orifice that enjoys being penetrated. Because it's so sensitive, many lovers find a finger, toy, or vajra sliding in and out of their rosetta (anus) extra erotic. With the proper preparation, it can release torrents of kundalini. For some, it's an intense way to play with domination and submission. That includes straight men receiving.

Maybe that's why there is a new backdoor-sex wave sweeping the world. Even Harvard University recently taught an anal sex class as part of their annual Sex Week. You both might find playing in this forbidden zone can be an amazing, orgasmic turbocharger.

Why?

Rosetta sex does require a learning curve. But once you get through it, it can produce a unique spiritual state of ecstasy. The opening, the canal, and the G areas are highly sensitive erectile sweet spots. The high density of nerve endings energizes powerful passion for both men and women.

Many women report that anal penetration feels totally different than vaginal sex. In addition to being a tighter fit when giving, men who learn to receive experience unique sensations. For both genders, it's a special joy that many lovers never get enough of.

Women crave rosetta sex when vajra's head directly impacts their G-crest while vajra's shaft rubs the lower sponge. The facts are similar for men receiving. The control center for the male orgasm, the prostate gland, is most easily impacted through rosetta sex.

It took Somraj years of practice before his rosetta comfortably welcomed penetration. Now he looks forward to it almost every time he makes love because of the intense and unique surges of kundalini that shoot through his entire body.

There are other advantages to rosetta sex. It's a reliable form of birth control. Because it requires a lot of communication and is one of the most intimate acts, it builds trust. It's a rare opportunity for assertive professionals like us to play at dominating each other. And it allows for the usually submissive partner to do the steering while the usually dominant partner simply follows.

Let's not ignore how titillating it can be for you to play in such an illicit erogenous zone. Many lovers who relish backdoor play feel like they are violating social norms and ignoring cultural taboos in the pursuit of new channels of ecstasy. If you're interested, consider how rosetta sex might help you let go of deep-seated inhibitions and unlock dormant energy pathways.

Agony or Ecstasy

Rosetta sex is not the safest or easiest form of lovemaking. The receiver has to really want it, and the giver has to take extra care. It requires even more warm-up than the average yoni and more attention to cleanliness. You need to use large amounts of lubrication and take it extra slow to avoid pain.

The rosetta is highly sensitive and prone to discomfort if abused or not opened properly. Unless you are cautious at first, it can generate more agony than ecstasy. The tightness factor requires even more care with first thrusts to avoid uncomfortable sphincter spasms.

Don't try to push through the body's instinctive self-protection mechanism. With enough pressure, you could force your way through the clenched doorway into the rectum. The initial traumatic spasm may disappear once the tissue has numbed, but it will likely leave a bad memory. This adds to the body armoring resident around the rosetta and likely prevents future appreciation of backdoor play.

Rosetta sex need not be uncomfortable or painful. If you give them time to adjust, the muscles relax of their own accord rather quickly. With repeated gentle practice, you can release the energetic armoring stored there. Once awakened, penetration will be welcomed, affording the chance to be transported to an altered state. That's how you maximize the ecstasy and eliminate the agony.

Backdoor Anatomy

Let's take a short tour around a man's backdoor anatomy as shown in figure 19, Male Rectum. The basic anatomy is very similar for a woman.

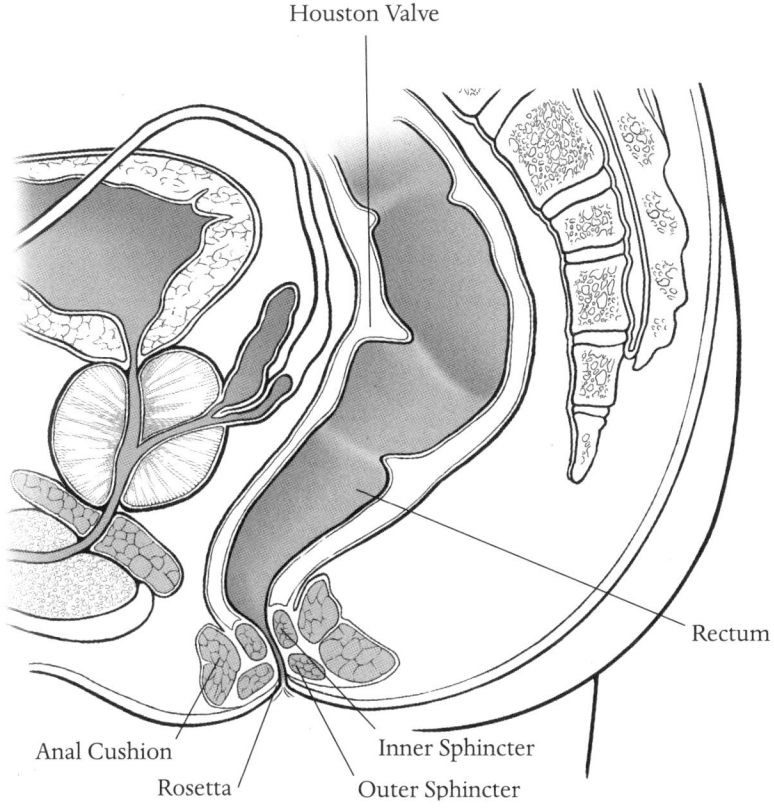

Figure 19: Male Rectum

Your rosetta is the external opening to the short *anal canal* at the bottom end of your gastrointestinal tract. The canal is a tube-shaped passageway, typically less than an inch long.

This little tube is guarded by two *sphincters* or ring-like muscles. It's lined with soft, delicate mucous membranes that contain a high concentration of tiny blood vessels and nerve endings.

This anatomy explains two things. First, your rosetta is usually pink in color unless irritated. Then it may appear bright red.

Second, it's highly sensitive. That's a result of having more nerve endings concentrated around the opening than anywhere else except the yoni and vajra. Because they're served by the same nerve pathways, this area can produce intense sensual pleasure.

The outside of your rosetta is puckered, due to folds of soft tissue, and populated by many hair follicles. Underneath the skin, it's surrounded by an *outer sphincter* that serves as the gatekeeper that keeps it closed until needed.

You can easily control rosetta's outer sphincter. You can readily contract and relax it when you choose. That is, of course, unless it's highly armored due to stored emotional baggage. Sadly, this is quite common.

The outer two-thirds of the tube is composed of the same soft, sensitive, highly expandable tissue that makes up the opening. The inner one-third is lined with mucous membranes. Like yoni, the outer part is more sensitive to touch and the inner part more to pressure.

If you penetrate the canal a quarter inch, you will discover the *inner sphincter* that overlaps the outer one. This internal valve is not easily relaxed since it's controlled by the autonomic nervous system. That's the involuntary nervous system that governs automatic bodily functions like heartbeat, digestion, and temperature regulation.

Going Deeper

Below the surface of the anal canal are three columns of tissue called *anal cushions*. They are connected to the inner sphincter and contain many blood vessels.

Normally, blood passes freely through the arteries and veins in the cushions. But if the sphincters are chronically tensed instead of relaxed, the blood can't leave. This is what causes discomfort, a stinging sensation, or pain from forced entry.

The good news is that you've got two gates keeping your waste products where they belong until you want otherwise. The bad news is that the internal valve, operating below your level of awareness, needs to be trained to relax and open on command. You can gradually learn to control the inner sphincter by inserting a finger or small toy and simply feeling.

A major drawback is that your inner sphincter responds to strong emotions like fear and anxiety. That means if you're armored down there, your backdoor shuts down really tight. And forcing your way in locks it closed.

Your *rectum* is the last part of your GI food processing system. It's around eight inches long and lies below your large intestine just above your anal canal. It's an elastic tube made of folds of loose, soft, smooth tissue.

When you insert a finger past the second ring muscle, you'll be able to feel things open up considerably. A few inches deeper into the rectum are several transverse folds of tissue called the *Houston's valves*. Pushing past them before they've relaxed also produces discomfort.

You'll also notice in figure 19 that the bottom of the rectum tilts toward the front of the body. Farther in it curves toward the back, and then, after a few more inches, it curves toward the front again. In other words, if you try to stick something in there that's longer, you'll run into this gentle S shape.

We include these details for one simple fact. Barging your way in may be stopped when you hit the Houston's valves or S-curves. If you proceed slowly, it will relax, straighten, and open for deeper stroking.

Preparations

Preparing for anal play requires more attention to detail than yoni penetration. Some fairly strong bacteria live inside your GI tract. As long as they stay there, they remain happy and so will you. But being the body's waste chute, these microorganisms aren't healthy for you elsewhere. That's why using a latex glove or condom is the safest practice.

Because anal tissues are delicate and don't provide much natural lubrication, they can easily tear and transmit STDs, or sexually transmitted diseases. In addition to barriers, use lots of water-based lube to minimize the chance of abrading the tissues and opening microscopic passages for infection.

How much lube should you use for rosetta play? A LOT, more than you think you need. To start, rub it all around with a finger. Then probe the opening and apply more lube up inside the anal canal. Even then, refresh it often.

After play, immediately wash everything that might have had any contact with anal tissues or fluids. Be extra careful of cross contamination to the yoni. The bacteria that live inside your rectum are unfriendly to vaginal health. That's why girls are always taught to wipe backward during toilet training so those bugs don't contaminate their yonis. You never want to transfer fluids, even lube, from a rosetta to a yoni by putting something in your backdoor and then back into the yoni.

Create a sacred space by gathering towels, wipes, gloves, condoms, and finger cots (latex finger condoms) along with sex toys. If either of you have interest in rosetta sex, discuss it during the partnering questions.

Rosetta sex doesn't have to be messy. We do it regularly without any problem. Just don't eat rich foods beforehand that might generate gas or gastric distress. Showering before and after is expected. Playing on bed-protection pads or towels gives you an extra level of comfort.

Still, sometimes rosetta sex gets dirty. If so, wipe off with the towels at hand and go wash. If you're wearing a glove or condom, pull it off from the base with your clean hand, wrap up the dirty parts inside, and throw it in the trash.

The good news is that the rectum is usually empty except just before you have to go to the toilet. Just to be sure, many anal-friendly lovers do an enema beforehand.

Opening Rosetta

If your rosetta isn't sexually experienced, build up to it slowly. The Tantric attitude, especially relaxing, is critical for this kind of adult play. If you can settle into your body, take responsibility for your own comfort and pleasure, and drop your goals and expectations, you'll have a lot more fun a lot sooner. That's why this practice can yield profound personal growth.

Most inexperienced anal lovers aren't really in touch with their inner derriere. Learning what feels good and what doesn't with fingers and toys is the best place to start. Spend a lot of time with solo anal play before involving your partner. This allows you to familiarize yourself with how your sphincters function and how to exercise some control over them.

Use the gradual insertion method to open your rosetta farther.

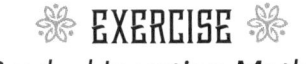

EXERCISE
Gradual Insertion Method

1. Start with a little finger before moving to larger ones and eventually two at a time.

2. Or buy a series of anal toys, commonly called *butt plugs,* of increasing girth. Pleasure yourself with the thinnest until it feels great. Then gradually increase the size. Make sure that the insertion at every stage feels good.

3. When your rosetta opens easily by yourself, thoroughly discuss the partnering questions with your lover. Get any concerns out in the open and decide how you'll handle them together.
4. When you're ready, ask your partner to repeat the fingering process. Drop any goals, agendas, time frames, or performance expectations before you begin.
5. Givers, be sure to ask permission before entering or changing anything that you're doing. As well, explain exactly what you're doing at each step, and quickly respond to any feedback.

Take your time with multiple practice sessions. If you go slow enough, you'll find that the ingrained tension is gradually dispelled. You may need to experiment to find a position that allows access and extended comfort for both of you. We often use extra pillows to support our backs, necks, arms, and legs.

Positions

Once you get going, jewel union through the backdoor isn't that different than through the front door. Most everything you've read so far applies to rosetta sex. What might be different is how much slower your first thrusts need to be and how often you'll need copious applications of lube.

Your sexual postures will require some adjustment. Here are a few suggestions:

Rear-Entry Postures

Most of the postures in the Rear-Entry Position are ideally suited for rosetta sex.

Side-to-Side Postures

Except when facing each other, postures in the Side-to-Side Position can easily be adjusted for rosetta penetration.

Man-Above and Man-Kneeling Positions

The Man-Above and Man-Kneeling Positions aren't the easiest for rosetta penetration. But rosetta sex can work if the receiver bends their legs and pulls their knees up to their chest or puts their feet on the giver's shoulders. The receiver's legs can be close together or wide but not down.

Woman-Above Position

During most postures of the Woman-Above, it's easy for a vajra to enter a rosetta, especially if she is leaning backward.

Sitting Position

In most Sitting Positions, with the receiver on the giver's lap, the receiver needs to rotate their pelvis up toward the giver. Or turn around.

Standing Position

Postures in the Standing Position are some of the most physically challenging for any kind of lovemaking, but if you're athletic, the receiver can lean over to expose your rosetta.

As always, find poses that allow for comfort, freedom of movement, and the best sensations for both of you.

Introducing Rosetta Sex

Receivers, relaxation is vital when engaging in anal play. Do whatever helps you both get into your body and out of your mind.

Givers, since this body part involuntarily tightens up at the drop of a hat, avoid undue physical or psychological pressure. Expecting, demanding, and forcing the issue may tighten, not loosen, the orifice you aim to visit. That's why introducing rosetta sex into your lovemaking depends on ample communication and collaboration.

Plan on an extended process over a series of sessions. One leading sex expert recommends easing your way in over a period of six days. It took us a lot longer. Only when you've developed a level of mutual trust and cooperation will you be ready to head into the backdoor.

Many women, like Jeffre, don't want anything inserted in their rosetta until they're very turned-on with lots of loveplay and yoni play (and after they've carefully discussed the partnering questions).

Being playful and easygoing demonstrates that the giver will be satisfied with whatever happens. You have to prove that you can be trusted and that you know what you're doing. It helps if you use the Last Stroke Technique introduced in chapter 3 about the Tantric attitude.

If you've both done your homework and his vajra is welcomed inside his partner's rosetta, be content with a few minutes your first time. Consider a few pleasant halfway strokes with no pain a roaring success. With patience, it gets easier and better.

Initial Rosetta Entry

Everything we've said about initial entry applies to rosetta sex in spades. It's up to the receiver's body when and if a vajra or toy will be invited in. The receiver must know that they're in control and the final authority on the depth, speed, and pressure of the stroking.

Givers, when you feel it's time, ask your sweetie before you do anything. Say something like "Are you ready for my vajra to enter your rosetta?" After ample loveplay elsewhere and being given permission, take charge of getting into a comfortable position. Start by sensually massaging all around the rosetta. Then gently apply some lube to the opening itself with a fingertip.

We both prefer lots of fingering before welcoming something larger.

Start penetration by simply resting vajra's well-lubed head up against the backdoor. Press gently and make your movements very subtle. If you're in a position where you can't see very well, don't be shy about tenderly using your fingers to feel around until you know exactly where vajra's head needs to be positioned.

Don't rush. There's no schedule, no agenda, nothing to do right now. The job for both of you is to relax, breathe, and feel. It's time to use everything you've learned about making vajra's first thrusts slow and gradual. Just like a tight or shy yoni, a rosetta needs to be opened like an umbrella to adjust to a vajra's presence.

Shower lots of sweet everythings. Check in often and instantly adjust what you're doing if the feedback you receive warrants it. You have to take it slow, pay attention to your playmate's verbal and nonverbal signals, and heed any feedback instantly. Add more lube anytime there's a hint it's needed.

When vajra's head is surrounded by rosetta's tender tissues and you hear good sounds, use a hand-assist to press your vajra outward. If you imagine a clock face with the rosetta at the center, you might try pressing at each hour's position. If gentle enough, this stretching should help relax the outer sphincter so that vajra's head penetrates a bit.

Try withdrawing ever so slowly and then reenter a few times. Continue these shallow first thrusts until vajra's head is gripped by rosetta's outer sphincter. If things are tight, a little shaking with your hand, pulsing with your sexual muscles, or vibrating with your hips may be in order.

When your playmate's rosetta relaxes and opens, try a slightly deeper stroke. If it's received well, repeat it. If not, pull back a tad or just hold still, giving the rosetta more time to unfold. Accept that this may be as far as you get.

If your initial thrusts are welcomed, descend deeper bit by bit. Keep lubing more than you think is necessary. Don't get carried away by violent thrusting yet. Shortly, you'll find your vajra up against your partner's inner sphincter. This is the one that's usually under involuntary control.

Maintain light pressure and take it ever so slowly again. Remember, don't push your way in. Let the second sphincter relax and the rosetta suck you through this second doorway like a vacuum cleaner.

Stimulating another erogenous zone can help accelerate rosetta's opening. Play with a woman's breasts, clio, or yoni. Play with a man's scrotum or vajra if you can reach.

❀ EXERCISE ❀
Rosetta Entry

1. Read this chapter together and discuss the partnering questions.
2. Begin with some loveplay and yoni jewel union to get thoroughly turned-on.
3. Once you have permission, find a comfortable sex position, put on a condom, and lube up.
4. Practice initial rosetta entry as described above.

A Nice Rhythm

Hopefully, you'll soon find yourselves stroking inside your beloved's rosetta not too differently than in a yoni. There will be more about that for both orifices in PART 5, The Valley.

It's important to realize the tissue between a woman's two canals—yoni and rosetta—is very thin. As a result, backdoor penetration that rubs and rams the spongy erectile tissue on yoni's upper wall is highly arousing. Some women find it's the easiest way to stimulate their G-crest.

Similarly, the tissue separating a man's rectum and prostate is thin. Rosetta sex is one of the best ways to pleasure a man's G-spot, his prostate gland.

Even after finding a nice stroking rhythm, you might find yourselves stumbling off track. Maybe the pumping is too vigorous. Maybe his vajra has hit the Houston's valves or S-curve in the rectum. Or maybe the sensations are too strong or weird for comfort. Do a check-in and adjust accordingly. Or wrap up your session and call your little adventure a success.

By the way, it's easy to accidentally switch orifices. Most yonis get thrown out of balance easily by anal germs. If this happens, there's no cause for alarm. Just take a short break and clean up before carrying on.

It can take multiple successful encounters of rosetta sex for a lover to become comfortable enough to totally surrender. That's why we view rosetta sex as a spiritual practice that releases armoring and builds trust. The next chapter about clearing energetic resistance and old traumas goes into this deeper.

Once you're past the armoring, the sky's the limit. The pulsing pleasure will indicate how well you're exchanging kundalini.

Summary and Action Steps

- Don't force your way into the rosetta.
- Learn to control the inner sphincter by inserting a finger or small toy.
- Use a glove, a condom, and lots of water-based lube.
- Play on towels or bed-protection pads.
- If your rosetta isn't sexually experienced, build up to it slowly.
- Spend a lot of time with solo anal play first.

- Use the gradual insertion method to open the rosetta.
- Plan on a series of sessions.
- Once you have permission, find a comfortable sex position.
- Practice with the Rosetta Entry Exercise.
- Be content with however far you penetrate at first.
- Experiment to learn how to hit your partner's G-crest or G-spot with rosetta sex.

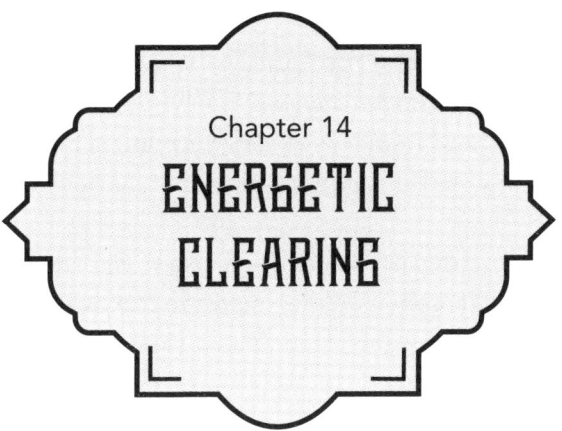

Chapter 14
ENERGETIC CLEARING

Tantra wasn't designed as a healing therapy to make you sexually whole. Still, lots of energetic Supernatural Sex gradually wears down energy blockages. Like the spring flood smoothing a streambed, running energy cleanses your channels.

In your native state, you get turned-on easily, your body pulses with kundalini, and your orgasms take you to an altered state of divine communion.

Yet, we all grow up with some sexual hang-ups and limitations. Our early fumbling attempts leave us embarrassed, frustrated, and wounded. Sex education is lacking, and we're bombarded with sex-negative messages. Far too many people, especially young girls, are subjected to sexual abuse and violence. This creates inhibitions against relaxing your body and enjoying your jewels.

As a result, most lovers don't look after their sexual fitness.

We urge you to replace your sexual fears, shame, guilt, or embarrassment with sex-positive beliefs through self-discovery, therapy, or energy healing. If your libido is weak, consider exercising more, changing your diet, and changing your medications. If menopause is an issue, see a physician who can prescribe bioidentical hormones or testosterone supplements. Regular self-pleasuring, ample loveplay, and frequent partnered sex are essential.

You can accelerate the process of opening your energy pathways with yoni and rosetta *clearing,* described shortly.

Body Armoring

Wilhelm Reich, an innovative psychoanalyst who built on Sigmund Freud's work, studied the flow of sexual energy in troubled patients. He proposed that many problems stemmed from *body armoring*. Armoring is the chronic tensing of soft tissues from stored energy traces lodged in the body by past traumatic experiences.

At rest, your sexual organs should be soft, pliant, and supple the way nature intended. But if you're armored down there, your muscles tighten and your tissues harden. This reduces the blood flow to your jewels, making it difficult to get aroused and feel pleasure.

When armoring persists, it deadens your sweet spots. This blocks feelings, sensitivity, and the free flow of kundalini. Armoring around the first and second chakras can create sexual performance anxiety, deep-seated inhibitions, painful intercourse, blocked orgasms, and frigidity.

Because massage therapists are restricted from touching anywhere near a client's privates, armored body parts are rarely touched in a way that releases the compacted energy to bring the tissues back to life. Sadly, many people just learn to live with armoring, coming to believe it's normal.

Various therapies have been developed over the years to release these energy imprints. Many of these healing methods are primarily "talk therapy," which isn't particularly quick or reliable. Fortunately, the acceptance of innovative forms of bodywork that stimulate blocked energy channels is growing. Certain physical therapists who specialize in pelvic floor function, for example, can work with you to resolve muscle and structural issues.

If you haven't found a way to awaken your orgasmic responses fast enough, we've had great success with the jewel-clearing processes that follow.

Yoni Clearing

Speaking energetically, a tense, tight yoni is armored by unwanted negative charge stored deep inside. In a sense, vajra's head can absorb yoni's tension during jewel union. With enough sexual play, it can channel away the residual emotion, release the tension, and unblock her nerve channels.

It's faster and more reliable, however, if you do repeated *yoni clearing*. Yoni clearing is a simple sexual healing process that uses loving touch to return full consciousness to all parts of a woman's yoni. To do yoni clearing, the giver slowly and gently massages around and inside a woman's yoni to reopen communication channels.[17]

The process identifies and targets blocked or dead areas to reopen yoni's innate stream of lifeforce. We call these points *hot spots*. Hot spots are armored tissues that store old energy. They can be tense, sore, hard, tender, painful, cold, or, as the name implies, burning. Sometimes the spot is numb to any sensation. When the energy is really dense, it feels like a hard nodule under the skin.

Both lovers have a vital role in yoni clearing. The giver sensually massages the receiver's body. Touching healthy tissue feels good. Contacting a hot spot produces some unnatural discomfort.

It's up to the receiver to report how things feel and guide her partner who then follows her lead. When a hot spot is identified, giver and receiver work together to create a circle of energy that releases the armoring. The real work of yoni clearing happens when the woman focuses her awareness where she's being touched.

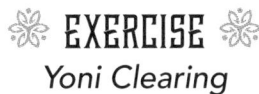

EXERCISE
Yoni Clearing

1. Center yourselves in the Tantric attitude.
2. Giver, start by slowly and sensuously touching the receiver all over.
3. Then move closer to the yoni and press lightly around the jewels to identify which tissues are supple and which are dense.
4. With agreement, use a wet finger to gently massage around outer yoni.
5. Gradually approach yoni's mouth and explore inside. Ask what the receiver is feeling at each step.
6. The clearing begins when the receiver alerts the giver that a hot spot has been contacted. The giver simply stops moving and holds with light pressure.
7. The receiver relaxes, breathes into the hot spot, and visualizes the compacted energy releasing on the out-breath. She may find it helpful to use

---

17. Margot Anand, *The Art of Sexual Ecstasy* (Los Angeles: Tarcher, 1989), 323–332.

orgasmic breathing while moaning, growling, or yelling to encourage the energy to move.

8. When the hot spot calms down, continue as above.

Sometimes the discomfort and tension seep away gradually in one or two breaths. Other times, she strongly reexperiences the pain for several minutes as the wounding releases. Sometimes strange images flash and disturbing memories resurface. We've seen dramatic emotional outbursts through tears, laughter, or screams. Often, both giver and receiver feel heat discharging or an electrical current running through the body as the trapped, negative energies dissipate.

Layers of Healing

Sexual healing is often like peeling an onion. You may need to repeat yoni clearing several times to remove layer after layer of distress. The faster you go, the more demanding, and possibly painful, it will be. But there's no rush. Cleanse her yoni a little at a time and soon you'll arrive where you've always wanted to be.

Though initially uncomfortable, running into a hot spot is a blessing. It provides an exact window into what needs to be confronted to free the unrestricted flow of sexual pleasure. After the compacted energy is released, pleasure, orgasm, and ecstatic states are much more easily accessed.

Some Tantric experts suggest the area that needs the most clearing is the G-crest. Others claim it's deep inside yoni's canal around the cervix and along the walls at the top. We approach yoni clearing with as few expectations as possible and just see what happens.

You may run into hot spots anytime you're making love that require you to switch from focusing on pleasure to healing and back again. Since this can be confusing for the receiver, we recommend you use the partnering questions to distinguish between sessions of yoni clearing versus free sexual play.

Years ago, Somraj was making love with an experienced Tantra teacher when his vajra impacted a deep hot spot. With a little shriek, she suddenly tightened up and tensed all over. He did the yoni clearing process except he used the head of his erection instead of a finger.

She was able to dispel the armoring with only a couple breaths, allowing them to resume jewel union. They came across a few more hot spots and banished them as easily. These brief detours allowed them to reach higher states of ecstasy without further interruption of jewel union.

Rosetta Clearing

Troubling emotions from life tension, work stress, and relationship conflict get stored in the surrounding pelvic muscles. The area around the rosetta is especially susceptible to armoring due to toilet training, sexual traumas, and punishment for masturbating. If earlier lovers forced their way in, the discomfort surely left a negative imprint.[18]

Like a divining rod, your rosetta is a highly accurate barometer of your comfort level in general. If your anus is locked, bolted, and shut tight, it won't enjoy any kind of attention, much less vajra penetration. Not only does it limit your physical sensitivity and prevent pleasure, but your rosetta will resist relaxing and opening.

There is a deeper layer of sexual healing that we call *rosetta clearing*. This process is nearly identical to yoni clearing except for the orifice it targets. For women, it releases different hot spots. For men, it's the best way to release armoring around the prostate.

Somraj has benefited tremendously from repeated rosetta clearing. When he first started his Tantra training, his anus was shut tight. Any touch was irritating and attempts to enter were painful.

But with a long program of short sessions over many months, he dispelled his backdoor armoring. Now anal penetration doesn't hurt in the least. Instead, it gives him great pleasure and releases waves of unique ecstasy.

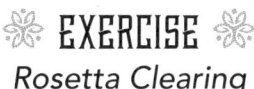

EXERCISE
Rosetta Clearing

1. Repeat the Yoni Clearing Exercise, instead focusing on the rosetta.
2. Giver, start by slowly and sensuously touching the receiver all over.
3. Then move closer to the rosetta and press lightly around the jewels to identify which tissues are supple and which are dense.

---

18. Margot Anand, *The Art of Sexual Ecstasy* (Los Angeles: Tarcher, 1989), 336–346.

4. With agreement, use a wet finger to gently massage around the rosetta.
5. Gradually approach the rosetta and explore inside. Ask what the receiver is feeling at each step.
6. The clearing begins when the receiver alerts the giver that a hot spot has been contacted. The giver simply stops moving and holds with light pressure.
7. The receiver relaxes, breathes into the hot spot, and visualizes the compacted energy releasing on the out-breath. They may find it helpful to moan, growl, or yell to encourage the energy to move.
8. When the hot spot calms down, continue as above.

Repetition of the above clearing methods is effective in addressing emotional and energetic traumas. But channeling kundalini doesn't depend on your physical condition. If you have physical limitations from an accident, illness, or heredity, you may still find that releasing armoring can free your channels to enjoy more pleasure.

Summary and Action Steps

- Replace your sex-negative beliefs with sex-positive ones.
- Improve your sexual fitness through exercise, diet, or different medications.
- Use lots of gentle loveplay; slow, tender lovemaking; or workable therapy to gradually melt body armoring.
- To accelerate sexual healing, use repeated sessions of the Yoni and Rosetta Clearing Exercises.

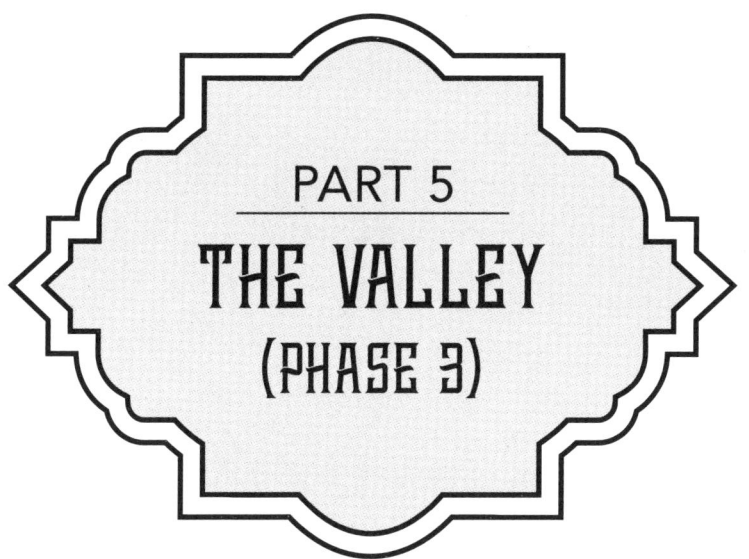

PART 5
THE VALLEY
(PHASE 3)

Phase 1, Loveplay, and phase 2, Initial Entry, have prepared you for the longest segment of Supernatural Sex. Phase 3 is the Valley, where you get to enjoy extended and rising pleasure.

PART 5 focuses on how to make jewel union last as long as you want. In the following chapters we'll look into using sexual strokes to hit sweet spots that release kundalini. Then we'll describe how to combine them into different schemes aiming for *sweet rhythms*. These are repeating patterns of sexual thrusts that produce continuing surges of pleasure.

To focus your partnership on maximizing the passion of your jewel union, the last chapter of PART 5 is about balancing power in Supernatural Sex.

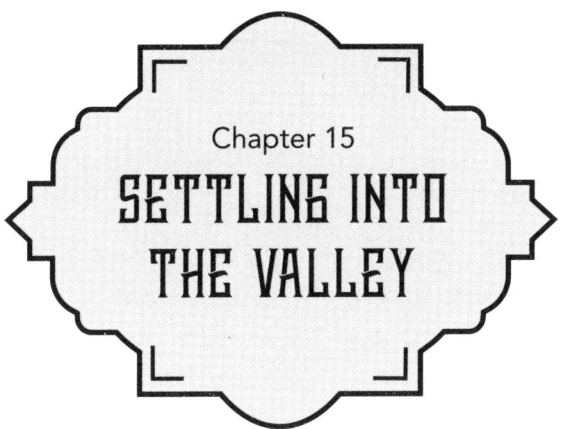

Chapter 15
SETTLING INTO THE VALLEY

Your goal in the Valley is to float as long as possible while generating ecstatic waves of kundalini. In its simplest terms, Supernatural Sex means finding that sensational point just before orgasm, getting as close as you can, and staying there as long as you want.

In the Valley, surges of energy recycle you back to the center instead of pushing you over the surrounding ramparts. The Valley resembles a snowboarder's half-pipe, a rounded channel with high walls. When your eruptions of pleasure propel you up the sides, you automatically slide back down for more.

You do that by orgasmic brinkmanship: edging, playing on the verge, building to multiple peaks, and relaxing without going over the top. (All things we'll get to soon.) This allows your sensations to become more and more intense without discharging much kundalini. Ultimately, when you get to climbing in phase 4, your orgasms will be fueled by much more energy, making them strong enough to spread though the whole body and repeat multiple times.

If one of you is rushing toward the Big O in the Valley while the other tries to prolong your play, the conflict will get in the way of your pleasure partnership.

To extend the Valley, start by adopting the Tantric attitude. Agree in the partnering questions to generate as much sexual energy as you can and see how long you can keep it going. Be in your body, not in your head, and relax into every sensation without any goal. Instead of tensing up, simply breathe and feel.

In the Valley, you cavort with sexual strokes and thrusting schemes, sweet spots and sweet rhythms. You explore and experiment until you find sensations you want more of. You concentrate on expanding your pleasure balloon to fill your entire biofield. You go with the flow and follow the energy.

An Example

Here's an example of playing in the Valley during jewel union. Somraj tried a series of slow, half-depth strokes with straight-in entry. On the out-stroke he pressed up against Jeffre's G-crest. She arched her back and let out a throaty growl as her sexual muscles contracted around his vajra.

Clearly that was working for her. Her yoni muscles were grabbing and squeezing his vajra tightly. She was reverberating like a bass drum beating a sweet rhythm up her insides. He felt it up his shaft and into his prostate as it spread throughout his pelvis.

When the vibrations dissipated after a few strokes, we tested out different postures, strokes, and schemes searching for another sweet rhythm. Her body asked for a few short, fast, shallow strokes around yoni's mouth and outlet, but that didn't produce much reaction.

When he thrusted deep and fast into her cul-de-sac, it made that drum beat again. She pushed back and wailed with delight. So, he repeated the stroke at the speed her hips requested. Twice more produced stronger reactions but they then faded.

He switched back to sliding halfway straight in and rubbing upward on the way out. The guttural moans returned but only briefly. Then he alternated deep, fast thrusts on her cervix with slow ones that pressed his shaft along her lower sponge. Wetness and heat engulfed him as her body vibrated with guttural moans. This sweet rhythm lasted longer so we milked it for all it was worth.

After a brief pause, we experimented some more. A simple steady rhythm that wasn't producing much erotic charge suddenly blossomed with strong energy bursts. But after a bit the fireworks evaporated.

In another lull a few moments later, we both felt a shock when vajra's head hit a spot up high and deep. Ahh, it was her A-spot. He held, pressed, and pulsed. Her hips started bouncing off the bed as she pushed back strongly.

He tried to follow her, but she didn't settle into one pattern. By slightly varying pressure, angle, and vibration, we finally found a rhythm that kept stoking the fire. She was writhing and whimpering while surges of liquid fire shot up his vajra and into his head.

Some of our grooves lasted for many minutes and others for only a few moments. But that was okay. We didn't have an agenda; we weren't going anywhere. We were just fiddling around having the kind of fun that our jewels excel at. It felt so good that all we wanted to do was wander around in the Valley searching for more.

Explore

The Valley is a relatively level pleasure playing field where your sensory fields are wide. Your energy body is getting bigger. The volume of sensation is expanding. To maximize your satisfaction, instead of aiming higher, focus on feeling more.

There's a whole smorgasbord of sensations waiting to be sampled. Some are electric, some are magnetic, some are loud and piercing, some are quiet and moving. It's like your bodies are getting massaged from the inside.

The more pleasure you generate, the more nerve endings are firing. You're not trying to blow the fuse on any one circuit, just activate more of them. You're so excited everywhere that there's no reason to reach higher when you can expand your pulsing pleasure balloon wider and wider.

One of the wonderful things about the Valley is that almost everything you try feels good. Searching for sweet spots is seemingly effortless fun. If a stroke or pattern doesn't evoke a strong response, you switch immediately. Just around the bend is another thundering starburst.

Because sweet spots don't last, keep adjusting your position, stroke, and points of connection with your beloved's body. Surf from one sweet rhythm to another as the waves of passion wash through you both.

In the Valley, you want the pleasure to last forever. There's little motivation to climb to orgasm.

Dancing on the Verge

Instead of pushing for maximum excitement all at once, concentrate on pumping your pleasure balloon full of orgasmic energy. That requires a skillful dance from one peak to another while you're on the brink of erupting. The popular name for this is *edging,* which means approaching orgasm but backing off before the point of no return.

We call edging again and again *dancing on the verge.* You don't just approach the brink of the precipice, you frolic there for minutes at a time. You float as long as you can at the rim where the ecstasy is most intense.

This gives you time to experience an endless variety of sensations that you don't want to miss. It's the pathway to an altered state of consciousness.

Dallying so close to orgasm makes your body shiver inside and out. You stretch your pleasure balloon and expand your capacity for pleasure. What felt like a ten on the ten-point scale of arousal a few minutes ago now feels like a six. You generate stronger and stronger currents of electrical sensation and rise close to a new ten.

Learn to savor the power locked within subtle energy sensations. Use the five cornerstones of ecstasy and orgasmic breathing to open your inner flutes and spread the juice around. By practicing more brinkmanship, you discover that you can take more, absorb more, and enjoy more pleasure.

While you learn, we encourage lots of communication. Agree on signals that you'll use when you want to go slower, faster, harder, or softer, or when you want to pause to savor and enjoy. Consciously practice reading your honey's signals and ask questions when you're not sure what's happening.

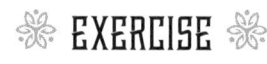

EXERCISE
Dancing on the Verge

1. Read this chapter together and agree on some cues to signal each other as to what you'll do.
2. Make love until one of you finds yourself close to a high peak of pleasure.
3. Slow or stop your motions, breathe, relax, and just feel the energy coursing through your body.
4. After a pause, repeat as many times as you want.

When you dance on this cloud of ecstasy, you'll naturally flow from one lovemaking position to another. A friend calls this seamless interchange of postures *lava lamping*. It also means moving vast tides of kundalini throughout your body and exchanging it with your beloved.

By the way, learning to play at the edge solves the common male pattern of premature ejaculation. For the average guy, that empties the reservoir, lowers the voltage, and depletes the energy reserves. He falls asleep leaving her unsatisfied.

When you learn to cling with one leg over the orgasmic ledge, the powerful buildup of lifeforces will unleash rare and wonderful sensations. When you dance on the verge, you'll feel the earth-moving power of orgasm continuously coursing through you, not just in the ten-second blaze of glory.

Summary and Action Steps

- Extend the Valley to generate as much sexual energy as you can and keep it going as long as you want.
- Go with the flow and follow the energy.
- Take your time and savor the whole smorgasbord of sensations.
- Don't push for maximum excitement all at once; concentrate on pumping your pleasure balloon full of orgasmic energy.
- To make the Valley last, practice edging with the Dancing on the Verge Exercise.
- Learn to savor the power locked within subtle energy sensations by focusing on the feelings, not on the climb to the Big O.

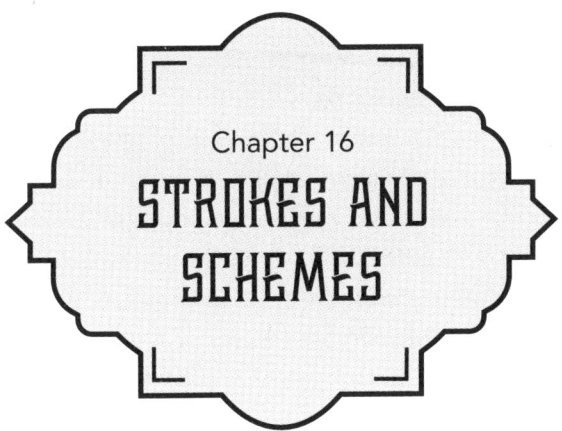

Chapter 16
STROKES AND SCHEMES

If you don't know where your and your partner's sweet spots are, your pleasure will be limited. Lovers who practice Supernatural Sex build the awareness and skills to best stimulate these hot zones with sexual strokes and thrusting schemes.

To target erogenous zones, you can vary your sexual strokes by changing their depth, length, speed, force, and angle of entry. Short strokes are great for targeting sweet spots directly. Short, shallow ones stimulate yoni's mouth, the outlet, and the lower sponge. By adjusting your posture, you can provide more stimulation to clio's crura (legs) and the V-bulbs on either side of inner yoni.

The first few inches of inner yoni are the snuggest and most sensitive. Short, shallow, gentle strokes are the safest bet for the first few thrusts during and just after initial entry.

The inner two-thirds of a woman's yoni responds more to pressure than friction. Longer thrusts can massage the deeper parts of the G-crest and the plexi (the nerve bundles) on either side of inner yoni when the vajra enters from left or right. Deep thrusts can powerfully stimulate a woman's womb, A-spot, cervix, and cul-de-sac. Stroking deeper allows you to crush your pelvic bones against each other with pubic grinding. Strong pelvic muscles help vajra's pulsing and bouncing and yoni's clasping and squeezing.

Since a woman's G-crest is actually the spongy, erectile tissue surrounding her several-inches-long urethra, there's no way to predict which spot will produce the most excitement. Experiment to see what feels best at each moment.

Relative jewel size affects how much force you can use. If his vajra is smaller than a yoni or rosetta, harder thrusting will probably be okay sooner. Otherwise, proceed more cautiously.

We recommend you play with a whole range of different paces during your lovemaking. Try fast or slow shallow strokes, then fast or slow deep ones.

Angle adjustment also allows a man to regulate his level of excitement. If you're getting a bit soft, enter shallowly at an extreme angle to increase the friction on vajra's sensitive head, crown, and frenulum. If you're getting too close to coming, try straight entry for a while.

One of our favorite techniques from the *Kama Sutra* is *churning*. That's when one of you rotates vajra's head with a hand-assist across the clio, vestibule, yoni's mouth, and rosetta. Inside, churning allows you to press sideways in all directions at various depths for variety and extra stimulation for a flagging erection.

It's not all up to the vajra owner. In Side-to-Side, Rear-Entry, Sitting, and Standing Positions, both can take the lead in shifting vajra's aim.

The woman can initiate many of the same things when she's riding on top, on her side, or when on all fours. If she raises her legs while she's on her back, it allows for insertion across the fourchette, the lower border of yoni's mouth. Or she can alter stroke angle by herself by raising just one leg.

All the above is also true for rosetta penetration. Since there are fewer sweet spots to target, thrusting into the inch or so of the anal canal is pretty straightforward. Once vajra's head is through the inner sphincter, only the shaft is squeezed.

Shallow, straight-in rosetta strokes seem to work best until the receiver fully relaxes. Because of the tighter fit, just about any kind of shallow strokes turn-on most vajras. The greatest advantage of deep thrusts into a rosetta is being able to more directly pummel a woman's G-crest or a man's G-spot.

Searching

While a vajra is sliding in and out at various angles and depths, it will contact energy bubbles and release dormant kundalini. You might be rocking back and forth with short, soft strokes and then suddenly a point that you've been sliding past seems hotter and brimming with sensation. Or stopping and holding suddenly sends out streamers pulsing with a delicious charge.

When you hit a sweet spot, narrow your focus and concentrate on milking it for all it's worth. At first, don't change what you're doing in any way.

Since the orgasmic energy generated by sweet spots comes and goes, stay with each one until it's depleted. If you find the response starting to wane, though, a subtle change in stroking can increase the energy stream momentarily.

You know you've settled into a sweet rhythm when a repeating pattern of strokes makes you swoon as kundalini discharges and spreads.

Stroking Schemes

A *stroking scheme* creates a pattern of sexual thrusts of different depth, length, speed, force, and angle during jewel union. A stroking scheme might look like a few shallow strokes followed by a few deep ones. Or a few light ones followed by one hard one. Or one really slow one followed by a series of fast jabs. Or alternating entry from side to side or high and low. Or going in slow and coming out fast or the reverse. Or entering one inch, then two inches, then three, and then withdrawing the same or completely differently.

Shifting gears with varying cadences introduces the excitement of surprise and awakens a wider spectrum of sweet spots. Stay on each sweet spot until the charge dissipates. When a scheme turns into a sweet rhythm, continue as long as it's generating sexual energy. When one brings you to a peak of pleasure, you might immediately repeat that or try another one.

Here's an example. Start by thrusting into her yoni three times at a depth of one inch. Then give her one deep fast thrust. Pause for a moment all the way in. Next, slide out as slowly as you can without completely withdrawing. Repeat the whole process with two-inch strokes before the single deep, extended plunge. Continue the scheme at a depth of three, four, five, and more inches.

Ancient Patterns

The simplest stroking scheme is called *karezza*, an Italian word that means *caress*. Karezza was first published in 1883 as the core practice of an open-group marriage in New York. Karezza starts with quiet meditation before some loveplay and initial entry. Then, for an hour or more, the man only moves his vajra enough to maintain an erection.

Many ancient Taoist, Tantric, and Arabian texts specified different movement patterns. The *Taoist Nines* detailed nine series of nine thrusts, each followed by a pause, totaling eighty-one thrusts. Another method required nine shallow thrusts followed by one deep stroke. A third begins with a set of eight shallow thrusts and then one deep. The next eighty-one sequences contained seven shallow and two deep. The scheme then shifted to six shallow and three deep strokes, and so on.[19]

Here are a few sample stroking schemes:

- Use a medley of ten steady strokes at one depth, speed, and angle, followed by another ten at a different depth, speed, and angle.
- Descend gradually starting with three shallow strokes, then three a little deeper, and so on.
- Alternate short, shallow strokes with long, deep ones, varying the speed as you go.

One of our favorites is the G-crest Rub, which starts with one deep, straight stroke. When she pushes back, slowly withdraw while angling vajra's shaft up her G-crest. Since G-crests are different and changeable, experiment to maximize her turn-on.

❊ EXERCISE ❊
Strokes and Schemes

1. Discuss the strokes and schemes you want to experiment with using the partnering questions.
2. Enjoy some loveplay until you're ready for initial entry.
3. Experiment with different strokes and schemes.
4. Discuss what you liked best.

Kaleidoscopic Rhythm

Our favorite stroking schemes organically develop without much conscious thought. If you follow the ebbs and flows of each other's energy, you'll invent new ones best suited to your bodies.

We often enjoy a *kaleidoscopic rhythm*. That's a continuously changing scheme without a repeating pattern. A kaleidoscopic rhythm shifts its "colors" in response to the ebbs and flows of energy at each chakra. In this kind of swirling

---

19. Nik Douglas and Penny Slinger, *Sexual Secrets* (Rochester, VT: Destiny Books, 2000), 206.

tempo, you frequently change gears. You start and stop as you shift position, angle, speed, and depth. Let your intuition guide you as you follow the morphing sensations.

We gravitate toward kaleidoscopic rhythms because kundalini loves variety. The same stroke only releases orgasmic energy for so long. What made you ecstatically vibrate at one point will soon go flat. Changing your pattern ensures that your jewels can't predict what's coming.

A clear advantage of employing the Tantric attitude is that it lets you drop your agendas, release your goals, and just go with the flow. When you continue to surprise each other, you keep your erogenous zones guessing. All you can do is get out of your head and into your body.

Habituation

Variety allows you to take your time to absorb, spread, and circulate kundalini. Sexual organs can only handle so much stimulation in a short period of time. Too much full-speed pumping numbs human tissues. This is called *habituation*, where an organism's response decreases after repeated stimulus.

If your sensitive zones get habituated, your sensitivity decreases. No matter how fast you pump, you feel less. Actually, the counterintuitive thing—slowing or even stopping frequently—works better.

We often shift our rhythm and take little breaks so that our waning sweet spots will have a chance to recover. Changing strokes and shifting positions helps prevent muscle discomfort that impedes free energy flow.

Sure, sometimes we love bouts of fast pumping. Yet we frequently cycle back to soulful, slow lovemaking. Going slow lets us charge our chakras, run energy, and feel more of each other's love.

Rushing almost guarantees you'll miss out on lots of pleasure. Draw out every stage of your coupling. Drop your rush toward the Big O. Keep changing your strokes and schemes. Slow down and smell the roses. Take little pauses that let your tissues renew. Focus on being in the pleasure of each moment. Savor every drop of sensual delight. Tune in to the subtler sensations of streaming orgasmic energy.

❊ EXERCISE ❊
Slow Variety

1. Make love as slowly as you can.

2. Anytime you feel a sweet spot or sweet rhythm bringing you pleasure, simply say "More."

3. Anytime you feel your sensations subsiding, say "Something different, please."

Whimsy

Intuition can help you discover your favorite stroking methods. Test and experiment, watch each other, and note what produces a "wow!"

After making love thousands of times, we find ourselves continuously reading how close the other is to orgasm and reacting accordingly. That might mean extending lovemaking to soar higher. Or, when the time is right, we might enlist our partner's help to explode over the top.

While Somraj was first learning Supernatural Sex, he discovered an interesting use of visualization. At first, his mind was flooded with distracting thoughts. But as he meditated more and the fog cleared, he noticed the occasional kinky idea floating by. An idea like pulling his vajra out and licking his beloved's yoni for a bit. Or rolling on top and thrusting his tongue deep into his honey's mouth in time with vajra's strokes.

At first, he didn't consider acting on these whims. When he started appreciating the divine wisdom at the root of these creative ideas, he started exploring the brainstorms. His whims generated unexpected variety, floods of passion, and juicy turn-ons that triggered delightful, sweet kaleidoscopic rhythms.

Whimsy is a state of mind where you let the lifeforce percolating through your body, mind, and spirit lead you. To apply whimsy, you must get out of your own way, not judge or dismiss these flashes of inspiration, and grab these fleeting gems before they disappear.

❊ EXERCISE ❊
Whimsy

1. The next time you make love, agree during the partnering questions to heed each other's whims.

2. Start by sitting across from each other in meditation.
3. When a loving, erotic, or kinky idea occurs to you, voice it and then act on it.
4. As you make love, continue shifting whenever one of you comes up with another whim.

Short Cycles

Supernatural Sex lovers ride the waves of kundalini in short spurts without going for maximum gratification all at once. You move for a while and then pause, savoring the sensations you've generated. The still moments let the energy swirl between you.

We call this pattern *short cycles*. Short could mean a few strokes or a few minutes depending on how turned-on or tired you are. Moving from one sexual posture to another naturally punctuates your jewel union with quick breaks. You could stay still during each pause or move slowly during the pause to keep the energy flowing.

Jeffre prefers short cycling because continuous pumping tends to make her habituated tissues numb. Somraj prefers short cycling because it lets him circulate kundalini to avoid coming. When we've settled into a sweet rhythm, short cycling lets us sink deeper into the sensations created and then recharge our batteries.

In a sense, short cycling intersperses vigorous lovemaking with little spells of the still style of karezza. If you're ultra turned-on, longer pauses let you calm down and pump up your pleasure balloons. If you're not super excited, longer active moments and shorter breaks serve you better. The more cycles you share, the more your arousal grows within each cycle.

❀ EXERCISE ❀
Short Cycles

1. The next time you make love, agree to try short cycling.
2. After a particularly intense passage, stop and relax for a moment.
3. Repeat 1 and 2 over and over.
4. Afterward, talk about how it made each of you feel and how you want to use short cycling in the future.

Summary and Action Steps

- Target sweet spots with shallow and deep, short and long, fast and slow, and hard and soft thrusts.
- Use churning for more stimulation inside and outside.
- Make the most of sweet spots and sweet rhythms by continuing as long as your tissues are bubbling with excitement.
- Experiment using the Strokes and Schemes Exercise.
- Use the Tantric attitude to create kaleidoscopic rhythms.
- Learn to avoid habituation with the Slow Variety Exercise.
- Practice following your erotic instincts with the Whimsy Exercise.
- Incorporate short cycling into your lovemaking with the Short Cycles Exercise.

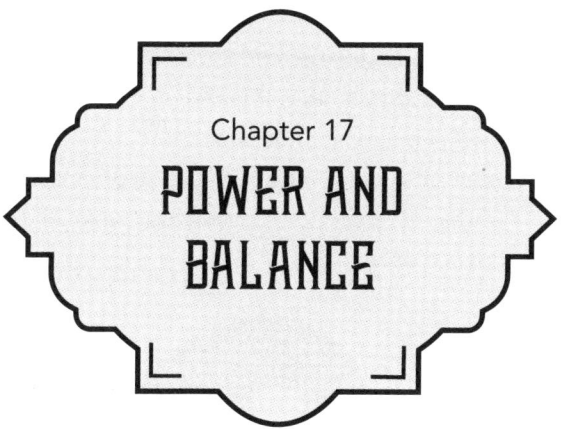

Chapter 17
POWER AND BALANCE

There are many different sexual styles. Some lovers prefer to come as quickly as possible, some prefer to dominate, some prefer to be taken. While many like it sweet, loving, and tender, others want it hard and even painful. Supernatural Sex is a partnered style rooted in the Tantric attitude in which lovers share power and ride the waves of ecstasy in sync.

Whatever style you choose, sexual pleasure is a moving target. A savvy vajra owner can discover the strokes and schemes that turn his partner on as the energy comes and goes. If he's getting feedback. Finding sweet spots and sweet rhythms takes cooperation from the receiver. That's why we say that synchronizing thrusts and patterns requires full, conscious collaboration.

Certainly, it's true that the giver's technique is pivotal. Timing, sensitivity, and communication are essential for a full-chakra connection.

When you play this way, you observe each other carefully, talk when needed, and adapt to each other's wants. You monitor each other's excitement and closeness to orgasm. You adjust to each other's mood, energy level, comfort, tiredness, body condition, jewel fit, and level of turn-on. You coordinate your motions so that your pleasure balloons fill and merge during jewel union.

In Supernatural Sex, you're continuously experimenting together. Chapter 17 describes this kind of partnership by presenting yin and yang roles, the receiver's responsiveness, and fantasy role-playing.

Yin and Yang

Carl Jung, a student of Sigmund Freud and father of transpersonal psychology, proposed that each of us has an inner self based on the opposite sex. Men have an inner female and women have an inner male.

The Eastern symbol of yin and yang in figure 20 demonstrates that within each of us is a part of the other gender. That's what the small dot in the middle of each side of the circle represents.

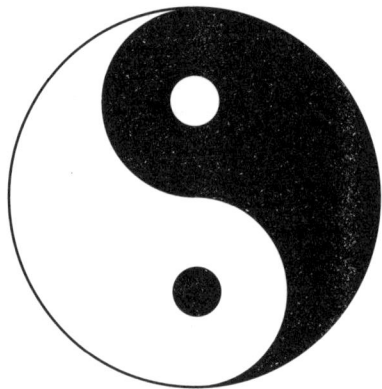

Figure 20: Yin and Yang

Traditionally, Western society has artificially separated our masculine and feminine qualities by discouraging us from developing the other's powers. You know that men are taught to hide their soft, feminine, pliant side and women are encouraged to hide their assertiveness, leadership, and personal power. For most of us, the dot inside each side of the yin-yang symbol is much smaller than the half circle around it.

Gender balance has always been a cornerstone of Tantric practice. Its earliest scriptures took the form of a dialogue between the god Shiva, representing the divine masculine, and his consort, Shakti, representing the divine feminine.

Shiva and Shakti

The qualities of each gender don't depend on your sex. Men and women operating from their Shiva side seek solutions, make decisions, act, and accomplish things. True masculinity rests in confident presence that focuses, witnesses, leads, and directs the course of action.

Shakti is more about energy and beauty, heart and love, nurturing and acceptance. Women and men who act from this essence revel in their senses, surrender to the flow of life, and bond with nature.

To dance with Supernatural Sex requires both polarities. Like the north and south poles of a bar magnet, opposites attract. If the feminine side of both of you is dominant, you might appreciate each other, but not much will happen in bed. If you both behave in a masculine way, you might experience more clashing than climaxing.

Your biological gender isn't as important as which role you're in, call it yin or yang, Shiva or Shakti, or, more accurately, which kind of energy is dominant at each moment. When you play the masculine role, take control. Assert what you want to give and receive, take charge of the proceedings, and move your partner's body when you need to. The masculine regulates the timing and leads in shifting from one fun thing to another.

We don't mean that you should be bossy and disrespectful. Observing, asking, and making suggestions is better than issuing military orders. Unless that's a fun game you've agreed to in the partnering questions.

Receiving

At first glance, givers of pleasure rely on their masculine qualities and receivers rely on their feminine. But there's more to it.

Receivers need to quietly lead, and givers need to listen and follow, too. Lovers in both roles must know their body and what brings them pleasure in each moment, a moving target for many. But if you communicate your desires of the moment, you can eliminate the confusion from the moving target.

Passive receivers rarely get everything they want in bed. Here are some things women can do to nonverbally control the action when receiving pleasure:

- Wrap your legs around your partner's thighs to pull his vajra in deeper.
- Grab his butt and hold him in place to pause his thrusting.
- When your clio is super sensitive, withdraw slightly. When it wants more, pull him closer.
- Reach for the lube bottle or ask for more when things are too dry inside.
- Squeeze your legs together when you want it slower or shallower.

- Spread your legs and push back when you want it deeper.
- Hold on tight when you want the vibrations engulfing you to play out.
- When you need a pause, stop moving and moaning or speak up.

Insist on creating enough intimacy to feel safe. Demand that your yoni or rosetta is fully erect before penetration. Take responsibility for making thrusts that contact your erogenous zones. Let your playmate know how you feel with words and nonverbal cues. Guide the action by sending clear signals about what you want more of and less of. Let the giver clearly know when you want help in going over the top.

Women, this applies to you when your hormones aren't calling you to easily sink into a sexual space. Take charge with your thoughts, focus on your desires, and remember your last ecstatic eruption. Or let your mind be consumed by a moving fantasy. Activate your love channels to drive your connection. For example, when she wants more clio stimulation, Jeffre stretches up the skin over her mound to expose her pearl.

You may consciously choose to surrender to your master of the moment, but you still guide what's being done to your body.

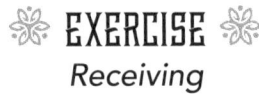

EXERCISE
Receiving

1. The next time you make love, agree with the partnering questions that whoever is receiving will be more assertive.
2. Receiver, ask for more of what you want and give more feedback in each moment.
3. Afterward, discuss how this power sharing worked for both of you.

Show Turn-On

Words are great for flirting, titillating, and sharing desires before you touch. Talking can bring you back together when you drift apart or off into your own private experience. However, too many words can put you squarely in your head and disturb your reverie.

We encourage you to show your turn-on with body language. Three of the five cornerstones of ecstasy—breath, sound, and movement—create a language all their own. Sighs, gasps, murmurs, screams, squirms, and shakes make your excitement evident.

Your body's response to arousal is natural. Blood rushes to your sweet spots making you hard or wet. Your breathing gets deeper, huskier, and faster. Erotic sounds erupt from deep in your throat. You roll your hips, spread your legs, and arch your back.

Let your body be a clear-cut turn-on meter when you reach for a sexual peak and pleasure streamers shoot through your body. Breathe deeper, moan louder, and shiver more as your arousal spikes. Shake, rattle, and roll. Exaggerate your primal responses. Even growl and flail.

A passionate lover who shows their turn-on is *responsive*. That means you don't physically hide your feelings by appearing cold, uninvolved, or inhibited. If you truly embrace the Tantric attitude, you won't be too "polite" to show your excitement. You'll be transparent, authentic, and real.

When you're in the dark about what's happening inside your honey, you won't be sure what to do next. You won't know what you did that created which feelings. You might be thinking instead of flowing kundalini.

Don't keep your passion a secret from each other. Use your body language to guide your giver.

Be as responsive as you can even if you're used to being quiet and still. Don't hold back the flood of passion that courses through you. Little by little, if you let go, you'll find your pleasure balloon expanding. And when your playmate sees, hears, and feels your turn-on, they'll get more turned-on, too.

Then, when the ecstasy in your beloved's body triggers a wave inside you, your honey will pick up on it. That will propel them to a peak. Which you feel and... Get the idea that being responsive keeps the continuous cycle going?

Giving

Were you raised, like Somraj, to believe that a real man always knows what to do? He got over that myth when he realized that supernatural lovers base their actions on connecting with their partner's energy. They discuss the partnering questions and continue talking. They ask permission before major changes. They check in and heed feedback. They monitor how it's going and adjust accordingly.

Certainly, givers draw on their experience of what was a previous turn-on. They creatively use sexual strokes and schemes, uncover sweet spots, and spark sweet rhythms. But in addition to leading, givers have to be pliant and receptive. They must be open to feedback. To pick up on subtle guidance, they need to let go of their egos, open their senses, and let themselves be led.

Unfortunately, many receivers have difficulty connecting with their sensations, especially from specific parts of their jewels. To counteract that, it's important for givers to tell their playmate what they're doing to them and where. We call this *labeling* your actions. Then they can connect what they're feeling with what you're doing to them.

Asking permission for initial entry is a perfect example of labeling before acting. You could say:

"Let's see how your yoni likes it real deep."

"I'm now going to do my best to give your G-crest/G-spot everything it deserves."

"How would you like a little vibrator on your clio while my vajra is busy inside?"

Labeling is particularly important during jewel clearing. Touching tense, armored tissues around the yoni or rosetta too quickly or hard can be shocking and sometimes painful. Be really clear with statements like "I'm putting my fingertip inside now."

If a giver keeps communicating like this, the receiver will become more aware of what's causing what feelings. They'll be less anxious about being shocked or hurt. Then they can creatively guide the giver to give them what they want.

Monitoring

Changes in your breathing, sounds, and movements can indicate whether you want it softer and slower or harder and faster. Since nonverbal cues are subtler than words, they don't do much good unless the giver is monitoring the receiver's reactions.

Monitoring means paying attention, watching, and observing. It requires being here and now, alert, and reaching out with your open senses. Givers monitor their partners by continuously reading their body for cues like these:

- **Breathing:** deeper, shallower, faster, slower, sighs, gasps, pants
- **Sounds:** murmurs, moans, cries, whimpers, wails, shouts, screams
- **Movements:** still, active, pulling, pushing, reaching, withdrawing, vibrating
- **Visual:** skin color, facial expression, body position

If you feel your partner's muscles contract while your jewels are engaged, you know something intense is happening inside. If you notice your partner suddenly becomes still and silent, you know something shifted and you might ask why.

Are her legs together or spread-eagle? Are his hands still or busy? Is his face flushed? Is her yoni wet and pink? Is his vajra harder, softer, or twitching?

With any luck, you've noticed partners crying out, curling their fingers and toes, arching their back, lifting their pelvis, tightening their butt, shaking all over, or forcefully grabbing you. Sometimes a man can feel his partner's heart beating and yoni or rosetta muscles spasming around his vajra.

If she pulls away, maybe you're going too fast or hard. Maybe it's too intense at this moment. Maybe you're hitting a tender spot that's not yet healed. If she pushes back and speeds her rhythm, maybe she wants it faster and harder right now.

Like other guys, Somraj used to ask his lovers, "Did you come yet?" There's nothing wrong with checking in if you're unsure. But if you have to ask, the answer is usually no. Sexual peaks of supernatural lovers aren't that subtle.

A Case

Let's say you're stroking slowly and deeply, almost pulling out completely before plunging gently as far as you can. You can tell she likes it because she's quivering and squealing in delight every time you descend.

After half a dozen strokes, you notice these responses are stronger when vajra's tip is being grabbed by the muscles around yoni's mouth. You follow her signals and shorten your strokes, thrusting shallowly without penetrating very far. She wails, "Oh my God!" so you know you've hit a good nerve.

After a few more strokes, she emits a deep groan, sighs, and relaxes into the mattress. You pause, following her lead. When you ask, "Did you like that?" from deep in her throat she says, "Yes, yes, yes! Can I have some more, please?"

It occurs to you that your last strokes were so good because your vajra was sliding across her G-crest. Consequently, you move your pelvis down a bit and aim vajra's head toward the upper wall of her yoni. After a couple of strokes, the strong reaction begins to subside.

Instead of forcing the issue and trying to prove yourself right, you notice the change and shift again. You move your pelvis up high and stroke vajra's shaft firmly against the upper vaginal wall. That makes her shiver and moan again, so you continue.

Receivers, you need to monitor your partner as well. Yes, you need to be aware of your own pleasure. But it's important to listen, watch, and feel where the giver is at, too. If he slows down, maybe he's getting too close to coming before you're ready. If he speeds up, maybe he's losing sensitivity or worried about getting too soft. As always, don't be afraid to ask.

❈ EXERCISE ❈
Synchronizing

1. The next time you make love, receiver, go overboard in showing your turn-on.
2. Giver, monitor your lover's reactions and respond accordingly.
3. To keep this monitoring process from putting you in your head, learn to move from head to body quickly. Practice by noting your own sensations and allowing yourself to sink into them.

Balance

Sometimes we put most of our attention on our playmate. For example, when Somraj's body shudders and he groans louder, Jeffre simply hangs on and enjoys the ride. When Jeffre's breathing changes and her body tenses, Somraj keeps doing what got her there in case she wants to explode over the top.

In those moments we have less attention on ourselves and more on our partner. But Supernatural Sex isn't selfless and one-sided. When you give, don't forget about your own pleasure.

Both of you need to achieve balance between giving and receiving. If your Shiva qualities are strong, develop your supple, receptive, sensitive, and vulnerable side without losing your masculinity. If your Shakti side is prominent, expand your vision, leadership, initiative, and teaching powers while retaining your femininity. More than anything, this balance defines the partnership of Supernatural Sex.

Instead of staying in one role all the time, play with interchanging yin/yang and Shiva/Shakti roles. Pursue what you want for a bit and then concentrate on your lover's pleasure. Alternate between taking the lead and surrendering to your sweetie's dominant side. By flowing between giving and taking, you'll surprise each other, touch unexpected sweet spots, open more channels, and exchange more ecstasy.

An effective way of balancing yin and yang in a relationship is by reversing roles. Whoever typically assumes the feminine position takes over the masculine, and vice versa. In the following exercise, one of you dominates the other for a predetermined period of time.[20]

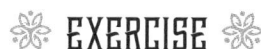

EXERCISE
The Shiva-Shakti Game

1. Agree that you will each play one role for an hour or an evening. You can do this in bed or anywhere and anytime you agree upon.
2. Whoever first plays Shiva takes the lead, requests services, and makes all the decisions.
3. The first Shakti politely follows and obeys everything asked of them.
4. When the time limit is up, share your feelings.
5. Switch roles.

Reversing Roles

After you try this outside the bedroom, play the game again during jewel union. The one who usually receives gets on top. The new Shiva directs loveplay, initial entry, stroking variables, and schemes.

The man on the bottom can still exercise a lot of choice about how his vajra moves inside his partner. He might lie still when he's close to coming or he might push his strokes upward deeper and faster if he wants more stimulation. Even though the lover on top is in charge, the one on the bottom guides the action, too.

---

20. Margot Anand, *The Art of Sexual Ecstasy* (Los Angeles: Tarcher, 1989), 257–270.

This is a great way for a woman to help a sensitive male lover last longer. Instead of going for it wildly after the first thrusts, she monitors how excited he is. When she senses (or he tells her) that he's close, she slows, giving him time to adjust and spread the energy out of his jewels.

Regardless of sexual position, a woman can use pompoir (yoni muscles that milk an inserted vajra, explained in chapter 10) to take charge. She can make him come when she chooses or relax when she wants the action to continue.

Domination and Submission

The fluid, spontaneous ebb and flow of power between two playmates keeps lovemaking fresh and new in each moment. Maybe that's why many adventuresome lovers are drawn to role-playing with dominance and submission.

It can be super arousing, especially for a powerful man who's in total charge of his life, to fully submit as the "bottom" while role-playing. And it can be really hot for a woman who's used to deferring to become the "top" or demanding master. The power play of dominance and submission can be accentuated by blindfolding the submissive, restraining them, or leashing and leading them around.

The surprising amount of energy released by dramatic role reversals like this comes from the inherent magnetism between masculine and feminine. The further from normal behavior, the stronger the erotic charge generated.

Playing top and bottom or dominator and submitter can't be done without a high degree of trust between partners. Mutual consent via the partnering questions is essential. Establishing boundaries and fail-safes makes the extreme more doable and the pleasure more resounding.

Fantasy Role-Playing

Another way to exchange power roles is to role-play fantasies that titillate you. Explore scenarios like threesomes, same-sex pickups, public sex, seducing dinner guests, and the ever-popular one-night stand.

Most of us have taboo dramas like these lurking inside our heads. They secretly titillate us because they're fueled by dormant kundalini. We suggest you experiment with what gets your sexual energy flowing and not judge another's kinks. Or your own.

Some fantasies may not translate well into role-playing in the real world, and that's okay. Just imagining the scene is often enough.

When consensual and regulated by the partnering questions, what might look like unrestrained domination from the outside is actually a true power-sharing collaboration. You just have to create a scenario together, each ask for what you want, talk about your concerns, and make your boundaries clear. It's also important to establish a *safe word* that gives the submissive the power to instantly stop the action.

Here's one way to use the partnering questions to negotiate a fantasy role-play:

Desires & Concerns
"I want you to pick me up in the grocery store, being all sweet and gentle. Then when you get me home, surprise me with handcuffs and tie me up. Cut my clothes off into shreds with a knife. I know you're skilled with a blade, so I'll trust you with that. And then tease me for hours until I scream for you to fuck me."

Boundaries
"You can do anything you want that doesn't cause me pain. My safe word is pumpernickel. If I say it, you must promise to stop role-playing and untie me immediately. Okay? If I say yellow light, it means I need to talk to you outside of my fantasy. Like maybe I'm thirsty or hurting or I have to pee. Okay?"

This is a safe way to explore your shadow side while having more fun. This often-hidden side harbors huge amounts of untapped energy. The possibilities for new sources of excitement are waiting for you right on the edge of your comfort zone. When your relationship is secure enough, give it a try.

Summary and Action Steps
- Develop and expose the energies of your opposite gender.
- Learn to lead when you're not in charge using the Receiving Exercise.
- Show your turn-on with your body language and don't keep your passion a secret from each other.
- Be as responsive as you can, even if you're used to being quiet and still.

- Base your actions on connecting with your partner's energy.
- Label your actions so the receiver can connect their sensations with what you're doing.
- Practice sharing power with the Synchronizing Exercise.
- Use the Shiva-Shakti Game Exercise to learn to exchange domination and submission.
- Role-play fantasies that titillate you.

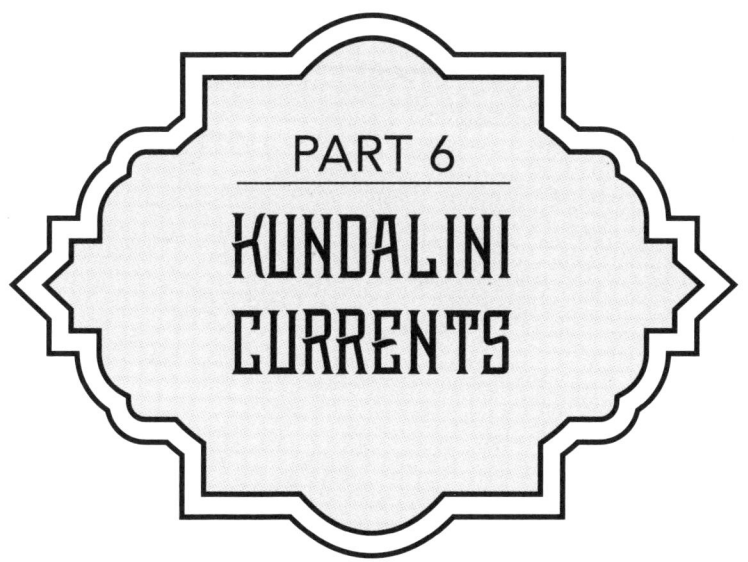

PART 6
KUNDALINI CURRENTS

We introduced sexual energy in PART 3, Kundalini, because managing erotic charge is the bedrock of Supernatural Sex. Now, in PART 6 we focus on exactly how you can direct and maximize currents of orgasmic energy.

The next chapters will give you the whole picture of opening energy channels, running and raising kundalini, streaming sexual electricity, hooking up hot links, exchanging orgasmic energy, and surfing from peak to peak.

One of the greatest things about jewel union is when you both feel the same thing at the same time. As you peak at a high level of excitement, your partner feels it in their body, too. That may catapult them to a state of ecstasy that you feel and react to. After alternating highs for a while, your ebbs and flows naturally synchronize. You start exchanging kundalini and sharing sensations.

One way this happens is by opening electrical circuits of passion between your bodies. Another is when you create energy circles that cycle kundalini between you. All these linkages can be physical, energetic, or both.

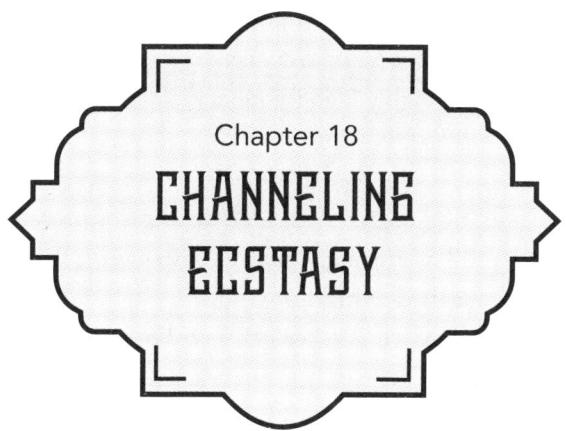

Chapter 18
CHANNELING ECSTASY

Ecstasy happens when your pleasure balloons are so filled with bristling kundalini that the energy spills over its normal borders to fully charge your biofield. We introduced this in chapter 10, The Five Cornerstones of Ecstasy: 1) being present, 2) the Tantric breath, 3) love sounds, 4) erotic movement, and 5) visualization.

Supernatural Sex helps you expand your sexual crescendos into wider, higher peaks of ecstasy. They cause electrical jolts and sonic booms that make every part of you reverberate with delight. And they can easily initiate multiple full-body orgasms.

In this chapter we want to aquaint you with the three steps of the pathway to ecstasy:

1. **Tuning in** to the subtle tickles in your body that sexual energy awakens, as explained in chapter 8, Energy
2. **Opening your channels** so kundalini can permeate your whole body, as introduced in chapter 9, Channels
3. **Running energy** to encourage its currents to freely flow until the sensations stream of their own accord, which is the theme of this chapter

Imagine what it feels like when that excitation making your jewels pulse infuses other parts of your body. That's what chapter 18 is about, the channeling of sexual ecstasy.

For sure, sexual friction plays a major part in this process. But you can't engage your subtle energy systems, anchored by your seven chakras, unless you involve your hearts, minds, emotions, and spirits. Then, when your biofields are throbbing with love and passion, every cell in your bodies will be so charged that they vibrate at an incredibly high frequency.

1. Tuning In

The path to sexual ecstasy begins with heightening your awareness of kundalini energy. It can be still or moving, dormant or dynamic. When erotic charge builds in your jewels, it's hard to miss.

You know you feel it when your crotch gets hot, hard, engorged, or wet. That's where goose bumps, shivers and shakes, and hot or cold flashes come from. Your brain contributes to the arousal process by sending nerve signals that release biochemicals. Strong emotions can initiate surges of hormones that turn on the flow.

But often the subtle lifeforce is hard to detect at first. When it's coursing through you during orgasm, there's nothing subdued about it. The more you can sense it when it's lying in wait, the easier you can awaken it into torrents of ecstasy.

To master your sexual energy, stay alert to even the wispiest tingles inside. Tune in to the fainter stirrings of kundalini anywhere in your body, such as tickles, prickles, itches, and buzzes. The more you pay attention to these tinges, the more easily you'll recognize the finer sensations of your sexual energy currents.

How to Feel It

The first and last of the five cornerstones of ecstasy, presence and visualization, are essential to feeling the faintest stirrings of kundalini.

Unless you're present in your body, you might not recognize these little sensations percolating, especially in unexpected places. Unless you focus your awareness and open all your senses, you'll likely miss the first tendrils of kundalini.

The last cornerstone, visualization, can help you tune your receiver. Imagining kundalini flowing in the bioelectric channels in your physical body will heighten your sensitivity to its delicate glimmers. Negativity or cynicism will undoubtedly kill any chance of sensing much.

Lifeforce energy vibrates many parts of your body. When you orgasm, everything is moving at top speed. But even at rest, your trillions of cells do their own little dance of respiration. The more excited you get, the faster more of them quiver. At intense peaks of ecstasy, they vibrate more strongly. At very high frequencies, these flimsy flutters turn into bed-rocking waves.

As you increase your sensitivity and open your channels, you become more able to feel this pervasive trembling when you're less turned-on. This is what you aim for.

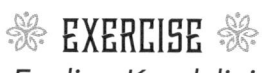
Feeling Kundalini

1. Find a quiet place where you won't be interrupted.
2. Sit still and watch your breath move in and out.
3. Then look inside your body with your mind's eye, slowly scanning from feet to head.
4. Notice the slightest sensation, where it is, and how it moves.
5. With your mind, imagine the sensation getting bigger and stronger, and moving.

2. Opening Your Channels

Ecstasy requires that you build erotic charge and channel the energy up your inner flute to all your chakras. This won't happen unless your circuits are open. When we say circuit, we're talking about your nerve channels, nadis like the inner flute, and spontaneous channels like hot links that you intentionally create. In their natural state, these energy pathways are open to the free flow of kundalini. But unless you keep them clean, life tends to clog them up.

The built-in resistances we all carry get in the way. Negative emotions form blockages in your nadis. This includes thoughts and beliefs that run counter to feeling pleasure. If a part of you hates sex because of painful experiences, intimacy conjures up the torment of failed relationships, or you still believe that some kinds of sex are a sin and you'll burn in hell for them, the free flow of kundalini energy that fuels sexual ecstasy will be impeded.

If you don't believe in the possibility of feeling kundalini or have doubts that you deserve pleasure, little is likely to happen. That's why opening to the flow of these subtle energies requires the Tantric attitude. Before you can be swept away, you have to uncork your mind to the undetected sexual lifeforces lurking inside. Start with the beginner's mind.

The body-mind defense mechanism against pain and trauma, body armoring may be the biggest obstacle to free-flowing kundalini. Here are some ways we successfully swept away our emotional rocks and mental boulders.

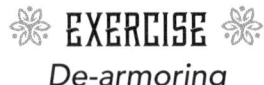

EXERCISE
De-armoring

1. Practice regular meditation with the Conscious Breathing and Self-Pleasuring Exercises in chapter 3, the Chakra Breathing Exercise in chapter 9, and the Orgasmic Breathing Exercise in chapter 10.
2. Engage in repeated yoni and rosetta clearing as presented in chapter 14, Energetic Clearing.
3. Dance and shake your body to free stuck energy.

Blockages

As you try to fill your pleasure balloon, you're likely to discover some energy gets lost. It's natural to leak lifeforce through any open orifices, referred to as *body gates*: eyes, nose, mouth, ears, jewels, and rosetta.

While opening these sense organs is sweet, it can cause kundalini leakage if you lose your center. Physically or psychically closing these body gates can slow or even stop the discharge. For example, focus your sounds inside instead of expelling lots of breath and lifeforce or keep your eyes closed when you need to build turn-on.

Resistance, muscle tension, and physical exertions also deplete you. Without relaxing all muscle tension, you'll unintentionally block the current through your inner flute. Of course, male ejaculation and explosive orgasm cause the biggest releases. On the other hand, some lucky women's orgasms don't deplete their energy and just keep going.

If your channels are clogged, constricted, or closed, rising sexual energy will be stopped or even bounce back down. This *reverse kundalini* flow can also be caused by physical problems like injuries, illnesses, a full stomach, constipation, female or male menopause, surgical removal of the womb and prostate, or simply a sore back.

While struggling to run energy during his early Tantra training, an instructor gave Somraj several network chiropractic adjustments for his locked-up lower back. They released a warm flow of energy up his spine. Thereafter, he could visualize and sense kundalini moving more easily.

If your channels are clogged, the above practices can help. If you have trouble sensing energy moving, try the following exercise.

❈ EXERCISE ❈
Releasing Blockages

- If your channels are at all blocked, get regular bodywork.
- Have your partner caress, blow into, tap, or strike your heart.
- Try this with the other chakras to release stuck energy.
- Also, thumping the sacrum at the base of the spine has been known to release congested kundalini.

3. Running Energy

Once you can sense kundalini at rest and open your channels, you can run it. *Running energy* means consciously moving and circulating it.

Before you learn to run energy, your lover's actions dictate where your sexual charge goes. That's often wonderful. But when you control it, you purposely direct the currents around your body to

- heighten or lessen the excitement in certain places,
- spread kundalini out of your jewels,
- expand your pleasure balloon to fill your biofield, and
- energize full-body orgasms.

Though its effects can be dramatic, sexual energy is more yin than yang. It's more fluid than solid. It's not something you can force. Like the spring flood, you can't stop it, only redirect its course. Therefore, we suggest you don't try to push or force it. Instead, relax into it and steer it with your intention.

Because most lovers can't go from zero to sixty by snapping their fingers, you need to jump-start the current flow. As your energy current builds, let go and surrender to the sensations of pleasure sweeping through you. Focus your inner eye, tune in to all sensory input, and consciously absorb the energy you feel into your pleasure balloon.

Like so many other parts of Supernatural Sex, running energy relies on the five cornerstones of ecstasy. When you get present and empty your mind of distracting thoughts, you can pivot your consciousness to visualize the energy moving within.

Untrained lovers usually pant or hold their breath as they get excited. Their muscles become tense and tight. The closer they get to the release of explosive orgasm, the more they shut off their senses and lose contact with their beloved.

Your go-to tool for running energy is orgasmic breathing. This is how you bring your mind, emotions, and spirit into harmony with your body.

Obviously the deeper you breathe, the more powerful the effects. Love sounds vibrate the tissues around your energy channels. Moving your body is also a potent energy activator. Rock your pelvis, undulate like a snake, and squeeze your pelvic floor muscles. Coupling all this with visualization magnifies the current.

Nonsexual Tools

Notice the above tools aren't directly sexual. Somraj vividly remembers the energy orgasm he had walking his dogs in the desert near Sedona, Arizona. The new Santana album was blasting in his headphones while the setting sun showered the sky with a rainbow of vibrant colors. The joy of his canine companions cavorting so freely plus the dynamic music made him dance uninhibitedly.

The impact of all these intoxicating senses started a trickle of pleasure up his inner flute. When he noticed the sensations, he used orgasmic breathing to focus on the little fountain bubbling in his torso. As a result, huge surges of sexual energy flooded his entire body during the thirty-minute hike. He felt all the manifestations of a *dry orgasm* without any jewel contact. That's an ecstatic peak with all the wonderful sensations of a male climax except for releasing semen.

This scenario highlights that the aim of Supernatural Sex is to run energy to heighten your pleasure and boost your ecstasy. We suggest you experiment with ways that help you move kundalini at will. Self-pleasuring is a great way to practice.

❈ EXERCISE ❈
Running Energy

1. With your hands or sex toys, build some fire in your jewels.
2. Use the Orgasmic Breathing Exercise from chapter 10 to expand your pleasure balloon.
3. While you touch your jewels with one hand, lightly stroke your lower belly and slide your fingertips upward to spread the energy.
4. When you gain some mastery of running energy solo, try it during jewel union.

Raising Kundalini

As we related in chapter 2, Energy Tools, excitement causes the dormant kundalini serpent at the base of your spine to uncurl and rise up your inner flute. Once you develop some skill in running energy, focus on raising it. We call this upward energy draw *raising kundalini*.

Spreading kundalini upward energizes your cells and cleanses your energy channels. Plus, channeling erotic charge upward is the essence of connecting sex with heart, mind, and spirit.

Since the chakras are intimately connected with your energy body, drawing kundalini up your inner flute allows it to charge your upper chakras and fuel higher levels of ecstasy as it pervades your biofield. This is how you pump your pleasure balloon full and activate full-body orgasms.

Your higher energy centers deal with power, love, voice, wisdom, and divine connection. The more energy you raise, the more spiritual your sex becomes.

Charging your fourth chakra by imagining the kundalini rising from your jewels up to your heart pours out a flood of love. Bring it to your head to energize your brain. Bring it up to your third eye to see visions and to your seventh chakra to heighten your spiritual wisdom. At the crown you may become one with God, Goddess, and the entire universe.

We learned to raise our kundalini by breathing up our chakras through the inner flute with the following daily practice.

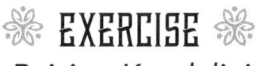 EXERCISE
Raising Kundalini

1. Sit in meditation for a few moments.
2. Start with the Orgasmic Breathing Exercise from chapter 10.
3. Focus your in-breaths on your first chakra.
4. Once you feel warmth or tingling in your jewels, visualize the energy moving up to your second chakra.
5. Continue visualizing the energy moving upward until it reaches your crown chakra.

When we first tried this exercise, we didn't feel much happen. Holding the fingertips of one hand on the perineum and tracing the upward flow with the fingers of the other hand helped us focus. As we breathed in, we imagined the air bathing the little sparks in our first chakras.

Eventually the image of a blooming flame rose up inside. We let the fire grow, expanding throughout our physical bodies. We pictured the current of kundalini as a glowing ball rising up our inner flutes to our upper chakras and brains. This pumped our pleasure balloons and expanded them to fill our biofields.

Flow Principle

In chapter 10, The Five Cornerstones of Ecstasy, we quoted the flow principle that states that "energy flows where attention goes." When you focus your attention on the parts of your body you want to heat up, it attracts lifeforce.

Erotic visualizations allow kundalini to flow more smoothly and strongly as if you were greasing the gears. Imagining sexual juice and electricity running will encourage it to happen. If you practice enough, all you have to do is visualize the tingly heat moving upward and you will feel it.

Don't expect the pictures in your mind to be as sharp as the real world around you at first. Accept whatever vague impressions appear regardless of their clarity, color, and relevance.

Like any muscle, the more you use it, the stronger it will become. This means you'll be able to visualize more easily and more solidly in your mind's eye. To strengthen your ability to visualize and run kundalini, simply picture the energy percolating and moving up your inner flute. Play with vibrant colors and familiar images like bubbles, geysers, winds, whirlpools, fireworks, or volcanos.

You can imagine a radiant white or golden ball of light emanating heat, red-hot streamers sending off electrical charges, warm blue rivulets massaging your tissues from the inside, or a shooting star blossoming up to your head. Also, try generating a fountain of love emanating from your heart.

Use whatever image helps tune your receiver to kundalini's quiet initial manifestations. Some people find this works better by focusing on the third eye behind the eyebrows.

Summary and Action Steps

- The path to sexual ecstasy begins with heightening your awareness of kundalini energy. Use the Feeling Kundalini Exercise to do this.
- Reach ecstasy by filling your pleasure balloon until it charges your entire biofield.
- To begin mastering your sexual energy, stay alert to even the wispiest tingles inside.
- Use presence and visualization to increase your sensitivity to kundalini.
- Open your energy channels with the De-armoring and Releasing Blockages Exercises.
- Dance and shake your body to free stuck energy.
- Learn to consciously move your kundalini with the Running Energy Exercise.
- Practice the Raising Kundalini Exercise until you can do it at will.

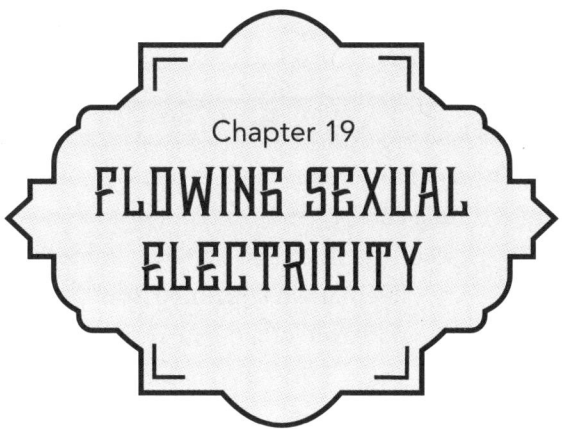

Chapter 19
FLOWING SEXUAL ELECTRICITY

Have you ever felt the meeting of your jewels was like plugging into an electrical socket? The more you channel sexual energy, the more it feels like an electrical current. These incandescent sensations include buzzing, sizzling, burning, and sparking. Flowing sexual electricity makes your organs quiver, your muscles shiver, and your bones pulse. The more current, the stronger the feelings.

Your jewels are powerful sexual electricity generators. The hotter and longer your sex, the more charge you create. The better your technique—or that of your lover—the more charge you create. The more you embrace the Tantric attitude and run energy, the more charge you create. The more connections you have at more chakras, the more charge you create.

Ever curled your toes while coming? Ever felt your knees quake? Ever felt your legs bounce off the bed? Well, that's the electricity descending. When your fingertips tingle, your scalp prickles, your teeth chatter, and your eyes roll, the charge is rising.

Sometimes it feels like an electric shock. Other times it's more like a heating pad.

Current

Like moving water, sexual electricity is a current. How wide and deep the river is and how much current flows determines how strong your sensations are.

When you only generate a little sexual electricity, you might not get wet or erect. With more current, you might find your skin tingling in a few places.

With top output, your whole body might shake with heat and vibrate with ecstasy. It's as if there's a conduit of sexual electricity from head to toe reverberating like a bass fiddle string.

Sometimes we can keep that electrical flow going for thirty to sixty minutes without stopping. Other times it surges for just a few seconds or minutes. We love it when a ball of sexual energy seems to erupt with an expanding blossom of sensation. It's like pleasure pyrotechnics exploding inside in different spots.

Can you feel the electrical sensations streaming from your groin and reaching your legs, chest, neck, and head? When you keep the current flowing for several minutes, you can actually sense the sexual electricity moving. Other times it feels like pulses and surges following your energy channels. From inside they look like streamers of fire that sometimes erupt into fireworks.

Do you know that an electric current creates *magnetism*? When you flow sexual energy and nerve signals pass to and fro from brain and body, it magnetizes your skin, nerve channels, muscles, and bones. This lifeforce not only energizes your passion, but also attracts your lover.

Voltage

Sexual current measures how much energy is flowing. Voltage measures how much pressure is behind the flow and how fast it moves. Have you noticed that sometimes a touch on your jewels is instantly electric? It's *sexual voltage* that makes you feel so sensitive. Almost like a spark jumping from your sex organ to your or your sweetie's hand, mouth, or jewels.

When your sexual voltage is high, it pushes the sensations faster and further around your body. Without enough sexual charge, your chances for multiple full-body orgasms are slim.

Sexual voltage tends to dissipate unless it's continuously reinforced. So most of the time when you're still during sex, your excitement gradually decreases. And the faster you move, the more intense the electrical charge you build—that is, until the spontaneous starts to stream spontaneously.

Now it's natural, as you first get turned-on, to push against the erotic current. Tightening your muscles keeps your pleasure balloon small and confines the electricity to a smaller space. This increases the voltage so your localized sensations are more intense.

That's partly why doing pelvic muscle exercises can strengthen your pleasure and orgasms. But when you tense up, you limit how much energy you can run and raise. As a result, only your jewels stay super excited.

Relaxing and visualizing the energy spreading upward tends to lower the excitement in your jewels. If you can generate enough sexual electricity to fill your whole body at high voltage, you'll almost levitate with passion.

When you're not very excited, keep your pleasure balloon confined to your jewels. Then, as you get more turned-on, relax and consciously open the valves. The electricity spreads out around your body. The bottom line is that someone who consciously works with their sexual electricity regulates where and how strong their turn-on is by adjusting their balance of tension versus relaxation.

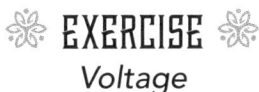

EXERCISE
Voltage

1. Self-pleasure until you feel your turn-on growing.
2. Keep your body still and your pelvic floor muscles contracted.
3. Feel the charge building in your jewels.
4. Relax and continue until another peak approaches.
5. This time use relaxation and orgasmic breathing to spread the kundalini upward.
6. Notice where your sensations are most intense from each experience.

Streaming

Streaming energy occurs when the erotic charge you've generated takes over, fills you, and flows where it will. Your kundalini is running of its own accord.[21]

Streaming feels like electricity sizzling, buzzing, and pulsing inside your energy pathways. That makes you tingle, vibrate, and shake all over. It can feel like fireworks shooting off, volcanos erupting, thunder booming, and lightning bursting inside. But mostly it seems like the electromagnetism that energizes intense passion.

Kundalini streams when you build up large amounts of electrical charge and let it go. It's like a tidal wave of ecstasy coursing through your body.

---

21. Margot Anand, *The Art of Sexual Ecstasy* (Los Angeles: Tarcher, 1989), 274–279.

You've undoubtedly experienced streaming when you've trembled in anticipation, felt hot flashes spread, or had goose bumps all over. The current makes your nerves twitter, the magnetism makes your muscles quiver, and the erotic charge makes your body undulate. This kind of streaming approaches energy orgasm.

When you easily stream orgasmic energy, your senses become immeasurably heightened. You'll experience powerful responses to subtle stimuli. When your energetic pathways are that open, you won't need much sexual stimulation to feel like you're coming.

Imagine what it will feel like when other parts of your body throb with the same excitation that makes your jewels pulse and throb. As you let the energy charge ripple inside, the natural vibrations will engulf you. That's a full-body orgasm.

Streaming while a vajra is stroking inside a yoni or rosetta is a truly ecstatic combination. But penetration isn't necessary when you can immerse yourself in the delightful shivering, shimmying, and shuddering.

Somraj remembers once swooning this way all night at a Tantric party in Las Vegas by holding a new, fully clothed lover close. It was sensational even without skin contact.

Streaming is a natural response to feeling ecstasy. As we explained, everything inside your body is in a constant state of vibration. When you get out of your own way and heighten your sensitivity, you become aware of these inner pulses as a subtle sense of vibration.

That's one key to learning to stream. First, you learn to notice the teeny tickles, welcome these new feelings, focus on the sensations, breathe into them, and let them take over. You turn your awareness inside and become more alert to incipient shivers, spurts, and spasms.

Visualization nudges the kundalini flow along. This is like tuning your receiver to pick up the subtler frequencies and then amplifying the weak radio signal to play at high volume. If the first energy twinges that you sense come from a sweet spot or sweet rhythm, they should be easy to follow. In this way, you plug into the lifeforces that are in constant motion.

Relaxation

The other key to streaming is, as we keep saying, relaxation. Tense and armored muscles, especially around the jewels and pelvic floor, will limit your free flow of kundalini.

If you resist the overflowing feelings that streaming creates, you'll tense up, pant, and pull away. You get caught in an internal conflict between reaching for and resisting pleasure. As the inner pulling versus pushing increases, at some point you'll lose control.

Instead of extended streaming, all the tension gets released in a big explosion. That interrupts the kundalini from rising and streaming throughout your body. You might feel really depleted or have to work hard to reawaken the turn-on.

Relaxing in a high state of excitement is how you clear the decks to allow streaming to flood all of you. What do you think would happen if you stayed relaxed and didn't fight the flood of sensation as you soared higher and higher?

First, off, you wouldn't spill all that delicious energy. This is true for many women as well as men who are prone to premature ejaculation. If you could relax with the waves of intense pleasure and avoid an involuntary orgasm, your body's streaming reflex would take over.

The surging currents of ecstatic electricity would fill your pleasure balloon and shoot throughout your body. You'd quiver, quaver, and quake with delight on and on. You'd feel the same sensations of jewel orgasm distributed throughout your whole body. That's an energy orgasm.

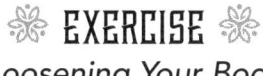

EXERCISE
Loosening Your Body

1. Prepare yourself to stream by loosening up your body with yoga or stretching.
2. Play some fast, rhythmic, electronic music that makes you want to move.
3. Stand with your knees slightly bent and bounce slightly in time with the beat.
4. Shake loose all parts of your body: head, shoulders, arms, hands, pelvis, legs, and knees.

The Five Cornerstones and Streaming

The five cornerstones of ecstasy (presence, breath, movement, sounds, and visualization) grease the wheels of streaming. Breathe slower and deeper through your mouth to fuel the fire. Let your body move and shake in rhythm with the first pleasure signals. Wriggle your hands and feet, flail your arms, roll your head, loosen your jaw, and let your whole body undulate as if you were a snake.

The sounding tool also strengthens the fledgling vibrations. Use your voice to oscillate wherever you feel the first stirrings of kundalini. Making sounds that express the sensation uses the physics law of resonance to amplify the vibrations.

One sensational effect of streaming is that the body shakes in delicious spasms of ecstasy, sometimes uncontrollably. When unexpected, it can be overwhelming. But when you have knowledge of what's occurring, you can revel in the pleasure of the experience.

We were personally involved in one such happening at a Tantra workshop with a longtime female friend. She had just left a highly confining long-term relationship that had caused her to suppress her free flow of kundalini. With just a little focused breathing, an inner dam burst, and she started shaking uncontrollably. Somraj hugged her to try to ground the energy until the instructor lay on top of her for fifteen minutes, which finally relaxed her.

As streaming becomes your go-to pathway, you'll find you can do it quicker, easier, and with less outside stimulation.

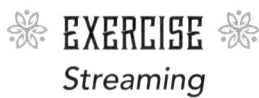
EXERCISE
Streaming

1. Do the Loosening Your Body Exercise to make it easier to relax.
2. Enter into jewel union until you feel a surge of sexual energy.
3. Relax, focus, breathe into the sensations, and visualize the kundalini blossoming.
4. Let the vibrations take over until you shake all over.

Summary and Action Steps

- The hotter and longer your lovemaking, the more sexual electricity you'll generate.
- The more connections you have at more chakras, the more charge you create.
- Constricting your pleasure balloon heightens your sexual voltage in your jewels. When you have enough energy, spread the electricity everywhere.
- To spread sexual electricity around your body, relax and open the valves.
- Practice the Voltage Exercise to learn to contain and expand your excitement.
- Energy streams when kundalini runs of its own accord.
- Use the Loosening Your Body Exercise to prepare for streaming.
- Practice letting sexual energy carry you away with the Streaming Exercise.

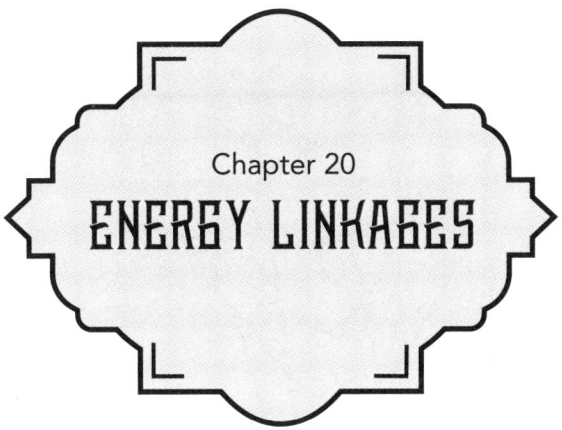

Chapter 20
ENERGY LINKAGES

We've made a lot of previous references to connecting your energy channels. In this chapter we're going to detail how to do that using hot links, passion circuits, and energy channels.

Hot Links

When you stimulate two sweet spots alternately or at the same time, you create a bioelectric linkage inside your body. We call this kundalini nadi a *hot link*. Whether by consciously running energy or involuntarily streaming it, the erotic charge tends to follow the circuit you've connected and amplifies your intimacy and passion.

Adding hot links during jewel union can be powerful, but you can hook them up virtually anywhere between other body parts. Figure 21 on page 192 shows a hot link inside each lover's body connecting their mouth and jewels.

Nonsexual actions like meditating together can open these linkages. Creating a sacred space is a form of hot link that piques all five senses. In face-to-face sexual positions, eye-gazing adds a delicious sense of romantic bonding.

Don't you get turned-on when your partner moans "Ahhh!" in your ear or murmurs "I love you"? When you speak your desires and have your feedback accepted when discussing the partnering questions, you open hot links.

Orgasmic breathing doesn't just turn your whole system on before lovemaking, but also opens hot links while coupling. The kundalini flow is especially potent if you're centered in your hearts and feel the love coursing between you.

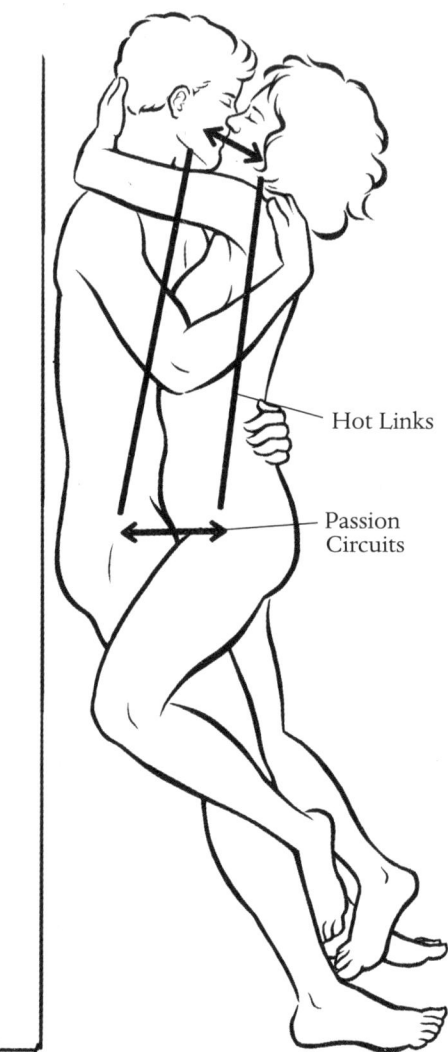

Figure 21: Hot Links, Passion Circuits, and Energy Circles

Sometimes the sensations at one end of a hot link are dominant while the other serves as a catalyst. Sometimes the roles reverse or both poles strongly sizzle. Because energy flows where attention goes, if a woman puts all attention on her clio during jewel union it will produce more pleasure there than if she's just concentrating on her yoni. And vice versa.

Even better is when your playmate is doing more than two things to you at once. For example, pulling a nipple and massaging a clio during jewel union creates a triangular circuit. Remember, there's no reason that any of your four hands should be idle.

Touching

You can create hot links with almost any body part when you generate sexual charge elsewhere. Doesn't a hand in your hair or a hug intensify a kiss? Or how about wrapping your fingers around the vajra or inserting them inside the yoni or rosetta while giving oral sex?

Sensual touch on a normally less-responsive place like a head, face, neck, shoulder, chest, tummy, side, back, foot, or butt cheek during jewel union can excite that area. Somraj once had a lover who was swept away by light caresses and baby kisses on her closed eyelids.

The *Kama Sutra* advocates extremes of squeezing, tapping, pulling, grabbing, flicking, vibrating, slapping, and scratching to inflame other body parts. The front and back of the seven chakras are especially sensitive on some people's bodies. Some zones, like the inner thighs, are so erogenous that caressing them alone opens a hot link to the jewels. Deep kissing makes Jeffre's yoni wet and sensuous back scratching makes Somraj's vajra hard.

Digital play—meaning fiddling wherever your fingers can reach—is a wonderful way to open hot links. Rousing another erogenous zone while vajra thrusts opens an energy channel that heightens the pleasure in both spots. For example, twirling a nipple during jewel union hooks up a hot link between the breasts and jewels. Jeffre still raves about the *thumbgasm* she once had from a lover sucking her thumb during lovemaking.

The vajra yoni-massage and hand-assist techniques we shared in chapter 11, Initial Entry, open hot links. Have you ever tried playing with a woman's lips, sensuously spreading them, stroking them, or squeezing them against your hard shaft? The touch provides extra stimulation for the receiver while it sends pleasure messages up the giver's arm.

Two of the most powerful hot links are between a man's prostate and vajra's head, and between a woman's G-crest and clio's pearl. Since most women need more than straight thrusting to orgasm, adding clio massage often adds the needed boost.

Also try alternating finger probes inside yoni with vajra's plunges. This stimulates her outlet and G-crest on and off during jewel union. Gently caressing, cupping, and scratching a scrotum with a soft hand adds some unique spice during coupling.

Though it's often a longer stretch, *postillionage*, French for rosetta play, adds an exciting and kinky dimension when a vajra penetrates a yoni. Depending on anatomy, an adept lover can insert a finger inside their partner's rosetta during yoni penetration or in her yoni during rosetta sex. Just be sure to use lots of lube plus a finger cot or thin latex/nitrile gloves and remove them or wash up before touching anywhere else.

Sometimes we play with our own sweet spots during jewel union to connect up hot links. Why not? Women, don't be too proud to massage your own throbbing pearl with a finger or vibrator. Men, try playing with your own scrotum or testicles, stroking the exposed part of your vajra, or massaging your own rosetta to add extra excitement.

The endless varieties of available sex toys accomplish the same connection. Jeffre's favorite is the *pocket rocket* vibrator, a three-inch-long cylinder that puts out quite a punch when applied to her clio. Many yonis and rosettas enjoy a dildo or butt plug while the other orifice is occupied.

Why limit your fun to digits? When your sexual posture allows, use your lips and tongue to kiss, lick, nibble, suck, or even bite all over each other's body.

Coupling

The more body contact you have during coupling, the easier it is to create hot links. Obviously, your sexual position and relative anatomies limit which erogenous zones you can access with your hands. The Scissors Posture is our favorite because we can both reach each other's private parts.

Face-to-face sexual positions like Man-Above, Sitting, and Standing allow for more skin-on-skin unlike Rear-Entry, Man-Kneeling, and Woman-on-Top. The Yab-Yum posture, with the woman sitting on the man's lap, is ideal for skin and energetic contact at multiple chakras at once.

Some sexual strokes automatically create hot links, which makes your jewels more sensitive. A deep thrust against a woman's cervix, for example, can stream energy between vajra's head and base or between vajra's head and testicles. Jabs into her A-spot simultaneously provide friction to her lower sponge, clio's legs, or V-bulbs.

Deep plunges with a high angle of entry allow vajra's shaft to vigorously polish a woman's clio, G-crest, and cul-de-sac. With lower penetration, the shaft can't help but rub her lower sponge while vajra's head pummels her A-spot. And deep backdoor sex certainly connects a woman's G-crest and sensitive rosetta opening.

Different strokes and postures also open hot links inside a man's body. When deep thrusts of vajra's head cause a woman's yoni muscles to spasm, they milk vajra's base and shaft like pompoir does. Long strokes inside his rosetta naturally connect his opening with his G-spot.

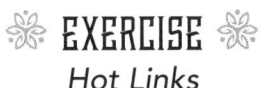
EXERCISE
Hot Links

1. The next time you make love, concentrate on opening as many hot links as you can.
2. Keep your hands busy exploring your sweetie's other sweet spots.
3. Shift to different sexual postures so you can reach new and different sweet spots.
4. Notice how energy spreads as you open hot links.

Passion Circuits

Have you ever felt a current of erotic charge when holding hands, hugging, or kissing? When you're present in love and conscious of energy, every caress can be electrically sensual. Even eye contact or feeling your honey's breath on your skin can cause sparks to jump between you.

Supernatural Sex goes beyond running kundalini in your body alone like hot links do. You can open nonphysical channels to exchange it with your beloved.

To some degree energy exchange automatically happens whenever you engage in loveplay and jewel union. The charge in your hands, sexual organs, and entire bodies tends to arc back and forth between you. That's what makes you feel each other's energy streams, blossoms, and fireworks.

When your bodies are pressed against each other, the energy can spark between your aligned chakras. That makes it easier to feel what's going inside each other's body.

Passion circuits are two-way channels between a sweet spot in each of your bodies that lets the sexual current run back and forth between you. Figure 22 on page 230 shows a passion circuit between the lovers' mouths and another connecting their jewels. The kundalini you receive mixes with your own and amplifies it. When you return it, the same thing happens inside your partner.

Slow and conscious initial entry is important in Supernatural Sex because you open the two-way energetic connection, the passion circuit, before the action heats up.

If you can imagine that a yoni or a rosetta is part of an old telephone operator's control board, tapping into a passion circuit is like plugging a vajra-headed cable into one of its sockets. When you plug in the sparking tip, you connect each other's erogenous zones to exchange kundalini.

Activated locales on vajra's head and crown open a circuit with yoni's or rosetta's sweet spots. Vajra yoni-massage links with her inner lips, mouth, outlet, fourchette, and lower sponge. Shallow strokes connect vajra with her G-crest, V-bulbs, and clio's legs. Deeper strokes connect vajra's head with her plexi, A-spot, cervix, and cul-de-sac. Pompoir couples yoni's sphincters with vajra's shaft or base.

Sometimes passion circuits open by themselves. Other times you must consciously connect them by intentionally running energy back and forth between you. Just don't speed up and go for broke in response to the intense cascade of sensation. Relax, move slowly, and breathe deeply into it. Let the kundalini do its thing.

A passion circuit is a self-reinforcing resonant loop. Your lover's feelings make you swoon. They feel your pleasure spike and it makes them swoon. And back and forth, inducing stronger sensations as you exchange energy.

Coming Together

One time we made love, initial entry released inner goose bumps and a surge of warmth inside both of us. As our thrusting intensified, Somraj felt a little electric shock of pleasure that made vajra's head swell and pulse. Jeffre felt the charge on vajra's head stream into her and started moaning loudly and bucking wildly. He felt the jolt of kundalini that made her yoni spasm. Her boosted turn-on flooded back into his body. The erotic charge grew into a cascade of sparks shooting back and forth between us.

These passion circuits really boosted our shared sensations. He visualized the high-voltage sexual charge in vajra's head sending bursts into her yoni. Her ramped-up passion made it clear that she was feeling the kundalini flares. The cascades of heat coursing up his vajra and inner flute made him vibrate in rhythm with her. The electrical streamers that he kept directing inside her triggered her orgasm, which in turn pushed him over the edge.

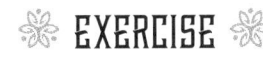

EXERCISE
Connecting Passion Circuits

1. Right after initial entry, focus on feeling each other's energy.
2. When the giver contacts one of the receiver's sweet spots, channel its energy with your attention into one of your own sweet spots to open a passion circuit.
3. Both visualize kudalini streaming back and forth in the passion circuit.

Energy Circles

After you've been in the Valley for a while, you often find multiple passion circuits activated between you. It's like a conference call with multiple cables plugged into different sockets in the switchboard. That makes your sensations grow and your pleasure balloons expand to fill your biofields.

When you connect two passion circuits, it creates an *energy circle* that circulates the pulsing kundalini in one circuit and out the other. The kundalini flows into one partner and returns through a passion circuit in the other partner. The circle is completed inside each body with a hot link as shown in figure 23.

You can open an energy circle by putting your hand on your sweetie's head, neck, heart, back, or butt while making love. Simultaneous oral sex, commonly called 69, is a clear-cut example. You can add even more energy by eye-gazing; touching foreheads; kissing; massaging a clio, breast, or scrotum; or playing with a rosetta.

Opening an energy circle to jewel union can dramatically boost your passion. If you first touch each other all over like we do, you'll activate several passion circuits. Then when your lovemaking starts, kundalini will already be sparking back and forth between multiple spots.

Scratching Somraj's back makes Jeffre's yoni wet. Caressing Jeffre's breasts awakens Somraj's vajra. Feeling each other's growing excitement turns us each on more. The more we connect energetically, the sooner we both get erect physically and energetically.

The power of such loops is why fondling during jewel union is so thrilling. Try touching your lover's belly, heart, or third eye—or any of the thirty-three secondary erogenous zones we listed in chapter 5, Loveplay—for example.

Face-to-face sexual positions easily open energy circles. Since liberated kundalini likes to ascend, the Yab-Yum Posture, embracing each other with one sitting on the other's lap, is ideal. With your eyes glued on each other, sharing breath with your mouths locked, and your jewels united, the orgasmic lifeforces have several channels through which they can cycle between you.

Since energy circles awaken more erogenous zones, they accelerate the spread of energy leading to full-body orgasms. Jeffre goes crazy with French kissing during jewel union. Somraj bucks wildly if a lover touches his head or feet while he makes love.

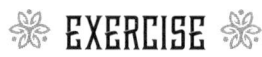

EXERCISE
Connecting Energy Circles

1. Right after initial entry, focus on feeling each other's energy.
2. Open two passion circuits as suggested above while you make love.
3. Both visualize kundalini streaming in one passion circuit and out the other.
4. It can help if you plan beforehand or indicate somehow in the moment which direction you each visualize the energy flowing.

Summary and Action Steps

- When you stimulate two sweet spots at the same time, you create a hot link.
- Verbal and nonverbal communication and kundalini currents to and from chakras can also open hot links.
- Keep your hands busy with digital play while making love.

- Trigger other sweet spots during jewel union with the Hot Links Exercise.
- Practice the Connecting Passion Circuits Exercise to exchange energy between sweet spots in each other's bodies.
- Create energy circles with two passion circuits that you each connect inside with a hot link.
- Use the Connecting Energy Circles Exercise to maximize your exchange of kundalini.

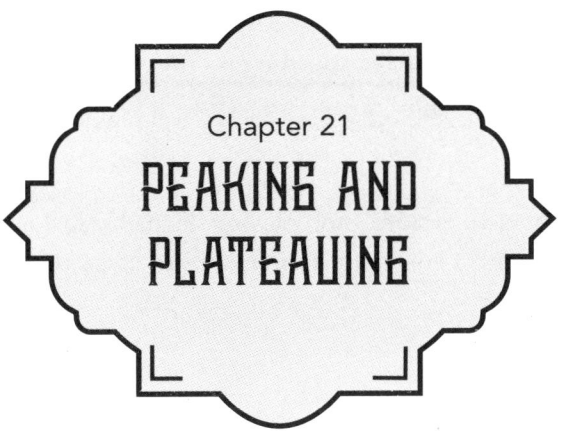

Chapter 21
PEAKING AND PLATEAUING

A sexual *peak* is a sudden surge of turn-on that rises to a high level and sharply drops back down. It's when your arousal suddenly spikes before dropping into a trough. The streaming unleashed by a peak of excitement is quick and intense like a mini-orgasm.

Sometimes soaring up to a peak is so exciting that it stretches your comfort zone. The unexpected flood of passion overloads your system, making it difficult to relax into the pleasure. The abrupt shock of electricity threatens to pop your pleasure balloon, wasting all that precious orgasmic energy before you're ready. The sharp, jarring jolt can numb you or drain your vital essence through energy release or male ejaculation.

If you know how to handle them, pleasure peaks can become your key to hotter and longer lovemaking. Somraj still remembers when our Tantra teacher instructed the class to pleasure themselves to a peak at least three times before coming. This exercise completely changed his sex life.

In the Valley, you build arousal and generate lots of sexual energy that you pump into your pleasure balloon. But sexual pleasure isn't a steady stream. Your level of turn-on ebbs and flows, comes and goes. You contact sweet spots, hook up hot links, settle into sweet rhythms, open passion circuits, and connect energy circles. When something feels good, you stay with it until it peters out and then move on.

The 5 S Formula

Use the 5 S formula to manage your surges of kundalini to hover just below the edge as you're peaking:

Stop

When you're about to explode, stop moving. Funnel sexual energy into your pleasure balloon with a couple of deep breaths to make your sensations subside.

Slow

When stopping works, soften your peaks by slowing your pace or pausing before your next stroke.

Switch

Next, practice switching by adjusting the depth, angle, speed, pressure, or pattern of your strokes. Or shift to a different sexual position.

Sound

Making love sounds spreads the energy as you rise to a peak. Using your voice releases a sudden surge of energy.

Spread

Spreading means running the energy out of your jewels. Consciously direct it upward and into your pleasure balloon using orgasmic breathing.

It's common to tense up when you're hit by a dense, heavy surge of kundalini. Unfortunately, tightening up blocks your energy channels. If you can't contain the lifeforce, you release all the energy in an explosive orgasm.

To learn to peak, practice solo first. Concentrate on ramping up, absorbing the sensations, and then floating for a little while before continuing. You do this by self-pleasuring your jewels with fingers, hands, or sex toys. Search for sweet spots and sweet rhythms, but without pushing for the Big O.

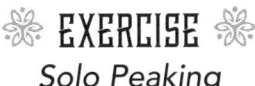
EXERCISE
Solo Peaking

1. Self-pleasure until you reach a peak.
2. Stop all motion and relax.
3. Next, practice coming back down past the precipice by simply slowing.
4. Experiment with switching the stimulation.
5. Add making sounds to release and spread the excitement.
6. When you're ready, keep your stimulation going at the top. Using the five cornerstones of ecstasy, spread the energy by drawing it up your inner flute.
7. Repeat the whole cycle at least three times.

Peaking Cycles

You have untapped reservoirs of potential kundalini that energize libido, sex drive, and sexual desire. You feel it strongly when you crave release. When you energize a hot link, passion circuit, or energy circle, the potential energy starts flowing.

The increased metabolism, firing nerves, shuddering muscles, deep breathing, and erotic moaning as you peak all require energy. Pausing occasionally with short cycles like we introduced in chapter 16, Strokes and Schemes, helps your body relax and your sexual batteries to recharge after these exertions.

Peaking is what drives short cycling. Thrusting to a peak and pausing defines one *peaking cycle*. Repeating the sequence is another cycle. Peaking cycles can last a few seconds or a few minutes. The pause might require a few seconds or longer.

At the start of each peaking cycle, you search for sweet spots and hook up hot links. When you settle into a sweet rhythm, your arousal spikes. You relax and surrender at the top, relishing the slide back down. Without unplugging, a short break of a few seconds seems the natural thing to do. But you don't have to completely stop moving during the pause between peaks.

Sliding down the back side of a peak can be delightful. When the bubble of sensations bursts at the top, it massages you inside and out with soft, energetic fingers. Likely, your body will vibrate as orgasmic energy percolates. Sometimes halfway down, a kriya (an involuntary jerk) is released, prompting more streaming. Or you can use a stroke or two to unleash any pockets of energy still hanging around.

During jewel union we don't recommend you push so hard that you go over the top, tire yourselves, or numb out. And don't stop so long that you lose your erection or misplace your turn-on. Starting up again with a twitch, shiver, or purposeful thrust is reflexive, which initiates another peaking cycle.

Surfing peaking cycles is different than other lovemaking styles. Many lovers like more nonstop coupling. (Sometimes we do, too.) Karezza and the Taoist Nines use different patterns. But whatever you prefer, you can add a pause between peaks to combine the best of both worlds.

An Example of Peaking

A peaking experience we had shows how we share leading and following.

A sweet rhythm catapulted Somraj to a peak close to ejaculating. In response, he slowed for a moment. Jeffre, who was grooving on the vigorous pumping, sensed the shift and relaxed into the flow. As she rested, kundalini started her hips slowly rocking until Somraj joined her rhythm. His lowered sensitivity allowed him to speed up again without losing it.

In the next peaking cycle, we plugged into another sweet rhythm, which spiked our excitement again. This time, Jeffre's body dramatically reacted with jerks, shakes, and shrieks of pleasure. At the summit, she stopped thrusting back against his strokes. He slowed, relaxed, and followed her down. When her vibrations and breathing slowed, he tested her readiness for another go around.

Sometimes she initiated the action by spreading her thighs, rocking her pelvis, pulling him close, or pushing into him. When one of us shuddered, moved, or uttered an erotic sound, we knew it was time to start another peaking cycle.

Orgasmic Surfing

Sailing from peak to peak is *orgasmic surfing*. You can use the big pulse of kundalini at the crest to propel you through the momentary pause to the next peak. Conserving kundalini is how you surf from pinnacle to pinnacle of pleasure. When you get in the groove, you can surf peaks for as much as an hour.

The first peaks in a series are often sharper and quicker. As you cycle up and down, your peaks reach higher and last longer. At the higher crests, the pleasure is more intense. The longer ones sustain the intense orgasmic sensations.

Sometimes diffuse crests develop over many minutes of stroking. These look more like rolling hills than sharp mountain summits. And some peaks are more persistent. You might find yourself plateauing or staying high without moving for many seconds or even minutes.

For the most part, the intensity and duration of pleasure peaks grow slowly. But the more peaks you surf, the more your pleasure balloon expands and your sensations spread, and the higher you'll ascend.

Sex becomes supernatural when you enjoy a long series of peaks.

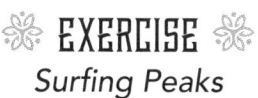

EXERCISE
Surfing Peaks

1. The next time you make love, agree to practice peaking cycles and surfing from peak to peak.
2. After you crest, briefly relax after the summit and see what you feel.
3. Use the streaming energy in the trough to propel you to the next peak.
4. Afterward, discuss how it worked and what you want to do more of.

Partner Peaking

Navigating from one peaking cycle to the next requires two-party coordination, which we call *partner peaking*. You need to get in sync with each other's ups and downs, peaks and troughs, changes and rhythms.

When one of you strokes, the other pushes back. When one of you slows, the other follows. When one of you speeds up, the other tags along. When one of you heeds a whim, the other changes their stroking pattern or sexual position to match.

Peaking together requires that you adapt to each other's preferences and idiosyncrasies. You help your lover peak by boosting the stimulation as they rise. To help them last, you use the 5 Ss to slow or still your movements, thereby lessening the stimulation near the top. You time your shifts so you don't interrupt their surges of pleasure.

As we said in chapter 17, Power and Balance, Supernatural Sex isn't completely selfless. It requires a balance of attention on yourself and your sweetie. You can't follow your partner's peaks and forget about your own for too long.

Because the average woman takes longer to get turned-on than a man, Somraj puts most of his initial attention on Jeffre's pleasure. Early in the Valley, he helps her reach a big peak after a series of growing ones.

He usually relaxes with her in the trough to feel the energy percolating between our bodies. Then he focuses on his own pleasure for a bit and crests himself. Naturally, that makes his arousal spike, and he soars over the top.

Alternating Peaks

This is *alternate peaking*. Once you're both flowing lots of erotic charge, one of you peaks while the other supports. Then you switch. You continue alternating back and forth. This looks a lot like leapfrogging. When you help your lover peak, the sexual charge floods your body. That makes you peak just afterward. When you're both open to it, this exchange of energy opens a passion circuit and may contribute to an energy circle.

It should be clear that alternating peaks can't happen if you're intent on pushing to climax as soon as possible. As well, to be able to start up again fresh, you both have to forget what happened before. In fact, you can't always expect to alternate one for one.

You both must tune in to NOW with the beginner's mind. That means reading your own level of arousal and at the same time reaching out with your senses to track what's happening with your honey. This is where the presence cornerstone is vital.

Givers, monitor what your partner experiences. Receivers, the more responsive you are, the clearer it will be to your partner when you peak. It's hard to miss when you let yourself quiver, shake, and vibrate.

Feeling what your beloved feels often activates *simultaneous peaking*. This is triggered when you get so turned-on by your partner's peak that you peak, too. And you open your energy channels to link up a passion circuit.

In a sweet rhythm, you gravitate to a speed that pleases you both. You ride the wave up and vibrate together. You relax in unison and let the pulses and blossoms of energy wash back and forth. When you feel the energy arcing between you, you don't change a thing.

It's as if your nervous systems are coupled while you're coupling. Your excitement streams into your lover's body and fills their pleasure balloon. You feel it while it happens, and it makes you soar alongside them. The ping-ponging kundalini choreographs you peaking together.

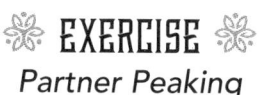

EXERCISE
Partner Peaking

1. Agree with the partnering questions that you'll practice alternate peaking.
2. Begin making love and when one of you peaks, the other supports and follows.
3. For your next peaking cycle, exchange roles.
4. Alternate back and forth for as long as you're having fun.
5. When you approach a peak, put some of your attention on sharing your energy with your partner.
6. When you support your partner's peak, put more of your attention on your partner's excitement.
7. When you start to feel each other's energy in your body, try to synchronize your peaks.
8. Afterward talk about how well you did and how you could get your peaks more in sync.

Plateauing

The Valley is characterized by peaks of roughly the same height and intensity. The orgasmic energy fills the Valley and permeates your biofield. As you leapfrog and surf together, you find that the steep ups and downs start to spread out. The highs last longer and the lows don't sink as far. As your erotic voltage increases, your peaks spread out, gradually morphing into *plateaus,* which are persistent peaks.

Plateauing means to maintain a high level of arousal without backing off. You move up to a high level of pleasure and stay there, enjoying it as long as you want.

As your pleasure balloon swells to fill the Valley, you can absorb more excitement and feel more passion. In this horizontal energy expansion, your mind and body eventually habituate to wave after wave of ecstasy. During a pleasure plateau, energy continues to stream through your body. The kriyas coalesce into stronger, lasting vibrations. The waves of passion become ecstatic.

When you decide you want more, you push your peaks of pleasure higher by drawing more orgasmic energy up your inner flute. The surges expand and intensify, shooting you higher. Your already charged chakras spin faster as currents of lifeforce pour through you.

Somraj recently had an experience of rosetta sex that offered a clear-cut contrast between peaking and plateauing. His initial pleasure peaks felt like detonating firecrackers, but they burned out quickly. When he amassed more kundalini, the same stroking caused expanding pyrotechnics that went on and on.

The knack of plateauing takes practice. Fingers are probably better to start with because they're more sensitive and allow better control.

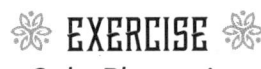

EXERCISE
Solo Plateauing

1. After sufficient warm-up, self-pleasure, letting your excitement build to peak after peak.
2. When you find yourself brimming full of kundalini, use orgasmic breathing to raise and spread the orgasmic energy.
3. At the next peak, keep doing what you were doing. Don't stop the stimulation completely as you relax and surrender into the sensations.
4. Keep the kundalini flow going to fuel the plateau.
5. When you've mastered plateauing solo, try it during jewel union.

How to Plateau

The limit to how much excitement you can contain in each moment depends on your capacity to absorb pleasure. If you tense up or explode, you'll have trouble plateauing.

But if you relax and breathe orgasmically, you can hover effortlessly as your body streams. The shaking vibrations sweep through you, washing your insides with life-giving passion. When you circulate the orgasmic energy up from your lower chakras this way, you simply let go and bask in the divine light that infuses your body, mind, and spirit. That's how you float on a plateau of pleasure.

Jeffre remarks that straight pumping is boring and makes her numb. She really loves to go slow, like pump, pump, pump, and then relax. She just lets the energy wash over her. Then a few more strokes and the orgasmic waves, little implosive orgasms, roll through her. By doing this over and over again and again, she eventually gets to higher and longer plateaus.

The longer one of your plateaus lasts, the more likely your partner will join you in a simultaneous plateau. Surfing through shared peaks and plateaus can go on like this for many minutes—sometimes fifteen, sometimes thirty, sometimes an hour.

During those summits, the feelings are so sensational that you'll find yourselves vibrating, undulating, and shrieking together. It's as if every nerve fires and every cell comes. You'll need all the heavy breathing you can handle to fuel your bodies.

Summary and Action Steps

- Manage your sudden bursts of sexual electricity by peaking.
- Use the 5 Ss, stopping, slowing, switching, sounding, and spreading, to learn to peak.
- Develop your peaking ability with the Solo Peaking Exercise.
- Make love in peaking cycles.
- Practice connecting your peaks with the Surfing Peaks Exercise.
- Help each other's turn-on rise and relax to coordinate your peaks.
- Pay attention to your own excitement as well as your partner's.
- Practice the Partner Peaking Exercise.
- A plateau is an extended peak where you maintain a high level of excitement without coming down.
- Learn to extend your peaks with the Solo Plateauing Exercise.

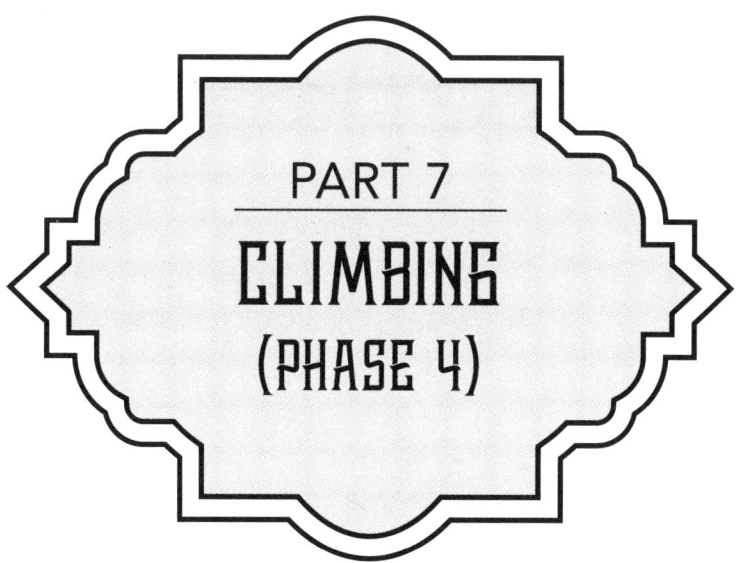

PART 7
CLIMBING
(PHASE 4)

Climbing in PART 7 will show you how to expand your repertoire of orgasms so you can ultimately float in high plateaus of ecstasy. That includes physical and energetic climaxes plus reaching the O-Zone, or orgasmic zone, when you're launched into orbit together.

In the Valley, you surf up and down peaks and troughs and float in plateaus of pleasure without going over the top. Then you make a conscious choice to climb all the way out of the Valley and reach for orgasm. You stop trying to extend your pleasure and shift to channeling all the energy into one or more sexual explosions.

Sometimes we float in a high plateau for a long while until we're propelled into the Climbing phase. Sometimes we're catapulted up to orgasm when the kundalini we've amassed spills over uncontrollably. But most often we each choose when we're ready to go for it, on occasion coming together.

When you decide to climb, you push your peaks higher and make the plateaus last longer. You increase the voltage and current of the sexual electricity in your passion circuits and energy circles. You use the overflowing reservoir of kundalini to create bigger, stronger, and longer orgasms.

Intense peaks and high plateaus are really just different kinds of orgasm. Though it's largely just a matter of semantics, let's look at the different ways to climax.

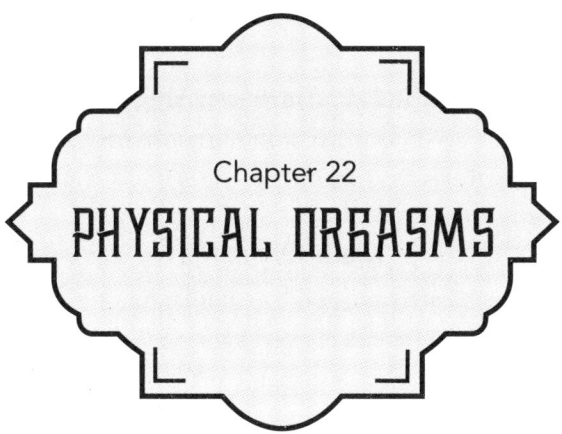

Chapter 22
PHYSICAL ORGASMS

When you grab the low-hanging fruit of the first chance to explode quickly, you might be denying yourselves lots more fun. On the other hand, when you extend your playtime with Supernatural Sex, you discover there are different forms of orgasms and different ways to achieve them.

We'll look into these in more detail beginning in this chapter, where we focus on physical orgasms. Men can enjoy a few of those while women, with more sweet spots, have more options. But don't worry guys, we'll end with multiple, blended, and simultaneous orgasms that allow you fully equal opportunity.

Explosive Orgasm

In chapter 2, Energy Tools, we defined orgasm as the sudden release of muscular tension in the jewels. We call these ordinary orgasms *explosive* because most of the accumulated sexual energy is discharged during the few-second blaze of glory.

Chapter 5, Loveplay, detailed what arousal does to your body. In an explosive orgasm, your metabolism, temperature, and blood pressure spike. Your heart rate doubles and your breathing rate triples. The outpouring of feel-good hormones wraps you up in waves of love and bliss. You may cry out, stretch your fingers, curl your toes, arch your back, lift your pelvis, tighten your butt, jackknife, or forcefully grab on to your lover.

Sometimes a man can feel his partner's heart beating around his vajra. Often you can both feel each other's sphincters contracting and pelvic muscles spasming. At the climax, the tension gets released in five to twelve rhythmic, involuntary contractions of the pelvic and anal muscles something on the order of ten seconds.

Then your metabolism and excitement steadily decline to the rest state before arousal is possible again. In other words, explosive orgasm is a charging-discharging cycle. Sometimes clearing out the pipes is just what you need.

Male Orgasms

Explosive male orgasms are triggered by stimulating one or more of a vajra's ten sweet spots. There are ten other sweet spots in the vicinity of a man's vajra that can activate orgasms, too. Most men equate orgasm and ejaculation. But as you'll see shortly, they are actually distinct.

Scientists say during an ejaculatory explosive orgasm a man's pelvic muscles contract ten to fifteen times within a few seconds. It's the intense and highly pleasurable pulsating sensations that make the physical release so delightful. When the pelvic floor muscles, prostate gland, and anal sphincter undergo repeated contractions, they produce the throbbing spasms that travel to vajra's head and farther.

Male ejaculatory orgasm occurs in two stages: *emission* of semen from the prostate, and *expulsion* that propels semen down the urethra and out vajra's head. When you can relax the emission contractions around the prostate, you can separate ejaculation from orgasm and enjoy a *dry orgasm*. This includes all the fun stuff without making a wet spot.

Dry orgasms are typically triggered by the same stimulation that causes ejaculation. Not only can you thoroughly enjoy all the powerful sensations of a physical orgasm, but you can do it multiple times. Somraj finds that a dry orgasm releases a fair amount of energy, which reduces his sensitivity and allows him to pump harder and faster right afterward.

A *male G-spot orgasm* is an inner one that's triggered by stimulating a man's prostate gland. Sometimes you can do this from the outside through the P-spot on the perineum. If a guy's rosetta is cleared, you can do this from the inside by inserting a gloved finger, erect vajra, or sex toy.

Because the prostate is orgasm central, male G-spot orgasms are deeper, fuller, and more intense than vajra-triggered climaxes. Somraj describes them as vibrating at a higher frequency. They may also trigger dry or ejaculatory climaxes.

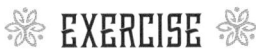 EXERCISE
Male Orgasm

1. Enjoy self-pleasuring until your pleasure balloon is brimming with energy.
2. At a peak, relax all your pelvic muscles to induce a dry orgasm.
3. When you're turned-on, try to induce a G-spot orgasm by pressing into the P-spot.
4. Use a finger or toy to directly stimulate the prostate to trigger a G-spot orgasm.
5. When you do ejaculate, pay close attention to the stages and sensations.

Female Orgasms

Women's outer orgasms are activated by the eleven sweet spots around the yoni, five on clio's various parts, and fourteen more inside. Women often describe outer climaxes as sharp and localized and inner ones as deeper, wider, and more moving. But your mileage may vary.

Sexologists claim the typical woman's orgasm lasts longer than a man's, twenty seconds on average. All the physiological responses listed earlier occur. The entire network surrounding the puffy cuff pulses in a variety of erotic rhythms. Her clio throbs, her pelvic and rosetta muscles spasm, her yoni muscles contract, the sponges all around yoni squeeze, her womb bobs up and down, and she experiences delightful tremors all over as everything vibrates.

The female orgasm is a complex process dramatically influenced by a woman's feelings about herself, her body, her surroundings, and, of course, her partner. In addition to the mechanics of sex, there are mental, emotional, relationship, energetic, and spiritual factors that influence how easily she can climax. In many cases, these are even more vital than the physical factors.

That's why most women need the hot links from a heart connection, a sacred space, and a sex-positive Tantric attitude to achieve their orgasmic potential. Supernatural Sex is perfect for women who want more.

Cliogasms

Though the outer yoni sweet spots have all been known to trigger a physical climax, the clio is arguably the most potent. Studies have shown that 70 to 80 percent of women need clio stimulation to reach orgasm.[22]

A *cliogasm* lasts from four to nineteen seconds. They are accompanied by rhythmic, rapid, one-second clenches of the outer third of inner yoni, the part nearest the opening. The bulbocavernosus and pelvic muscles tighten and pulsate as do the womb muscles and anal sphincters.

A cliogasm creates an intensely pleasurable feeling of pelvic fullness, body tension, and scrumptious waves that build to a sharp peak. While many women say that cliogasms are rhythmic, intense, and extensive, others claim that they're shallow, superficial, and localized. Some say they're sharper and faster than those from jewel union alone.

If a woman's clio isn't close to yoni's mouth, it's unlikely that a stroking vajra will stimulate it. A recent study[23] found that clios lie from 0.62 to 1.75 inches from the urethral outlet at the top of yoni's mouth. Those whose clios were more than one inch away didn't get enough friction to push them over the top. We've heard this amounts to 90 percent of women.

That's one reason why we're such strong advocates of adding hot links that involve the clio in jewel union.

Yonigasms

Exciting the sweet spots inside a woman's yoni can activate a *yonigasm*. On average this takes longer to trigger than cliogasms, typically between twenty and forty minutes.

Yonigasms tend to be longer, deeper, and more emotional than those of the shorter cliogasm variety. Some women report that they commonly last forty-five seconds, while others say they can go on for many minutes.

---

22. Lizette Borelli, "The Sex Moves Women Want: Clitoral Stimulation Helps Female Orgasm, Study Finds." Newsweek.com. 9/21/2017. https://www.newsweek.com/sex-moves-female-orgasm-relationships-dating-669154.

23. Ally Hirschlag. "Why Some Women Orgasm Easier Than Others." SheKnows.com. 5/6/2016. https://www.sheknows.com/love-and-sex/articles/1120927/why-some-women-have-better-orgasms.

Some women say that yonigasms create constant waves that spread out strongly from the deep pelvic and uterine muscles. It's like a pressure slowly building that explodes and expands from deep inside. Others describe them as lower in the body but less intense than cliogasms.

Sexologists are still studying yonigasms, but it's likely that any of the inner sweet spots can activate them. There's no doubt that a woman's G-crest is one of the most powerful orgasmic triggers.

A *G-crest orgasm* is often accompanied by deep contractions that feel as if the uterus is pushing down toward yoni's opening. Women say that G-crest orgasms are longer, stronger, and more intense than cliogasms. They report wave after wave of contractions making them shake, shudder, and vibrate.

We believe that deeper yonigasms are usually more fulfilling and more emotional. That may explain why they require more intimacy, cooperation, and trust. If you don't feel safe and powerful enough to unleash your kundalini, you aren't as likely to get there.

Female Ejaculation

Have you ever found that the female jewels are wetter at times? While level of turn-on could explain the difference, ejaculation may be the cause. Though many modern professionals are dubious, there are ample references to female ejaculation from ancient Tantric texts, Greek physicians, Dutch scientists, and indigenous cultures.

Sexologists estimate that 10 to 54 percent of women ejaculate when properly stimulated.[24] This means emitting sexual fluids distinct from yoni lubrication. Some dribble, some gush, some downright squirt. Mostly this happens during orgasm, but some women can ejaculate at other times when really turned-on.

Jeffre enjoys this added release when she's orgasming, and other times, too. Believe her when she says, "It's a truly ecstatic experience that you don't want to miss out on!"

Not understanding what happened, many women and their lovers have been revolted, thinking they expelled urine. But that's not the case. Female

---

24. Streicher, Lauren, MD. "Science Says Yes to Female Ejaculation." EverydayHealth.com. 8/25/2016. https://www.everydayhealth.com/columns/lauren-streicher-midlife-menopause-and-beyond/female-ejaculation/.

ejaculate, or *amrita,* is a mostly clear fluid that resembles male semen. Though the exact physiology has yet to be completely documented, it's apparent that amrita comes at least in part from the urethral sponge.

Various forms of stimulation, notably on the G-crest, have been shown to produce a climax accompanied by female ejaculation. Probably many more women would naturally ejaculate if they didn't avoid the sensation of having to urinate that's produced from intense G-crest stimulation.

If you're intimate with your partner and willing to give it a try, you may well be showered by these sacred secretions. Just don't make it a goal that creates pressure.

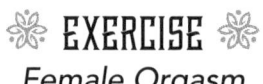

EXERCISE
Female Orgasm

1. Self-pleasure to reach a high level of yoni erection.
2. Experiment with yonigasms and cliogasms.
3. To practice ejaculation, fully empty your bladder and play on towels.
4. At a peak, strongly push out with your yoni muscles.

Multiple Orgasm

If men and women keep going after one climax, they can experience *multiple orgasms.* That's a series of climaxes with a brief pause between. After one explosion, excitement naturally dips down a bit for a moment. But if you resume stroking, you may trigger another climax at the same level as the previous one.

Multiple orgasm is typically easier for a woman whose arousal doesn't diminish as much as a man's. Many women are naturally multiply orgasmic, especially those who enjoy ejaculating. While repeat male ejaculatory orgasms are rarer without a long break, men can also repeatedly come if they've learned to separate orgasm from ejaculation.

Enjoying multiple orgasms is more than just a physical technique. When you release a surge of energy, your desire for more decreases. If you've nearly emptied your pleasure balloon, you'll have to push yourself to rise again.

The more kundalini you've pumped into your pleasure balloon, the easier it is to have a series of repeat performances. Surfing from peak to peak and plateau to plateau without an intervening explosive climax is a surefire way to activate multiple orgasms.

Blended Orgasm

A *blended orgasm* for both men and women is triggered by stimulating two or more sweet spots alternately or at the same time. That makes the explosion bigger and stronger. And it's why hooking up hot links is so powerful.

Dealing with multiple sources of pleasure is both the delight and challenge of blended orgasms. You may well receive more sensation than you're accustomed to. Can you pump so much kundalini into your pleasure balloon so quickly?

Blended orgasms require that the receiver focuses on two places in the body at the same time. Unless you stay relaxed in the moment, it's easy to get distracted, tense up, or resist. You have to drop into a meditative no-mind condition and surrender to the natural forces within your body to let the pleasure sweep you away.

Giving blended stimulation is a major challenge as well. The giver has to pay attention to the responses of two or more body parts while maintaining two different rhythms. It's like listening to two radio channels while trying to play two musical instruments in tune with the two music channels simultaneously.

Without a lot of experience, a lover can't give each separate channel the attention it deserves. To tune in to the ebbs and flows of your beloved's energy takes confidence, total presence, and a clear head. That's why we've found that blended orgasm takes lots of practice for both giver and receiver. But it sure is fun and rewarding when you get the hang of it.

Simultaneous Orgasm

Is sex supposed to culminate in a *simultaneous orgasm*? That's when you come within a few seconds of one another. For example, a woman has an inner orgasm during jewel union while a man ejaculates.

Sharing the sensations amplifies them at multiple chakras. Undoubtedly it can be one of the most satisfying conclusions to lovemaking with your beloved. Unfortunately, coming together is not as common as romance novels and movies would lead you to believe.

While the average man takes just a few minutes to ejaculate, the average woman takes twenty minutes or more to cross the finish line. That's why timing is a major challenge. The pathway depends on him lasting long enough and you both becoming expert at spurring her orgasmic triggers.

Though not every peak is an orgasm, the better you are at peaking and plateauing together, the more likely you'll be to explode simultaneously. Opening passion circuits and energy circles that harmonize your ebbs and flows makes it much more likely.

Coming together is obviously a partnering process. If you've gotten good at communicating and collaborating, you're partway there.

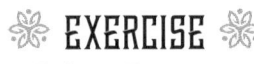

EXERCISE
Other Orgasms

1. After your first explosion, push yourself to have multiples.
2. Try stimulating two sweet spots at the same time to trigger a blended orgasm.
3. Practice the above by yourself first. When you know what works for you, practice together.
4. Finally, practice timing your climaxes so you can orgasm together during jewel union.

Other Ways

There are many more types of orgasm and ways to trigger them. And some talented lovers can think themselves off.

When kundalini pools in other places in the body, they can become orgasmic sweet spots. When you hook up hot links from erogenous zones to different areas, you can activate otherwise neutral tissues. When you run energy to various chakras, you can spur a wide spectrum of pleasure crescendos.

As well, what you do during and immediately after your lover's physical orgasm is critical. When a lover relaxes into the orgasm and kundalini is still swirling inside, *aftershocks* are quite common. These are short vibrations, surges of pleasure, and captivating contractions that erupt on the downside of the explosive peak. Sometimes they're triggered by slight movements, deep breaths, or simply remembering how good the climax was.

The most sensitive parts of both gender's jewels become hypersensitive right after coming. Jeffre has taught Somraj to be especially careful not to touch her clio when she relaxes after a Big O. Vajra's head requires the same hands-off and mouth-off approach for most men after ejaculating.

Consequently, you don't want to resume sudden vigorous thrusting right away. But a slow, short stroke or Kegel pump can trigger some wonderful waves of pleasure spreading throughout your bodies. Take it easy and let the subtle surges swirl and settle on their own. You may be able to encourage several short spells of aftershocks this way as long as you pause between them. And if you choose to push through the trough after a bit, you can trigger another orgasm.

Also, don't abruptly pull away after an explosion. It's great to maintain the intimate connection where your hands or bodies are touching. It feels wonderful to carefully place a hand around vajra's shrinking shaft or a palm over yoni's mound and mouth.

Keeping your energy channels open and flowing as the orgasmic forces subside is a sweet and loving way to show your gratitude for what you've co-created. Passionate lovers who are brimming with kundalini can set off energy orgasms much later just by replaying the experience in their minds.

Summary and Action Steps

- Explosive orgasm is the sudden release of muscular tension in the jewels.
- Male explosive orgasms result from stimulating one or more of a vajra's ten sweet spots or the ten others in the neighborhood.
- When a man learns to relax the contractions around his prostate, he can separate ejaculation from orgasm and enjoy a dry orgasm.
- A male G-spot orgasm is an inner one that's triggered by stimulating a man's prostate gland.
- Practice with the Male Orgasm Exercise.
- Women's outer orgasms are activated by the eleven sweet spots around the yoni, five on clio, and fourteen more inside.
- Women describe cliogasms and yonigasms as quite different.
- With practice, a woman may well learn to release female ejaculation.

- Experiment with different kinds of climaxes with the Female Orgasm Exercise.
- Experiment with multiple, blended, and simultaneous orgasms with the Other Orgasms Exercise.
- Carefully trigger and enjoy aftershocks.

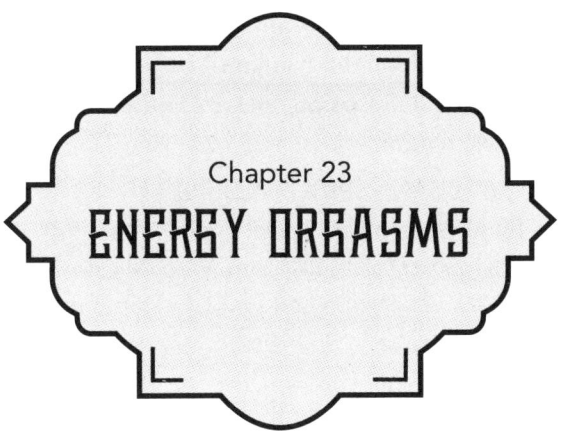

Chapter 23
ENERGY ORGASMS

When Somraj began studying Tantra, he complained, "Don't try to persuade me to give up ejaculating. I love coming and plan to continue well past one hundred." That was before he understood why any guy would want to postpone explosive orgasm.

Coming is glorious when the time is right. But if you take your time and fill your pleasure balloon, you and your sweetheart can stay orgasmic as long as you choose. When you learn to surf from peak to peak, you'll prefer to float in the high plateaus beyond the verge.

If you don't discharge like a lightning bolt and expend the fuel that feeds your passion, you'll naturally experience energy orgasms instead. An *energy orgasm* is a plateau of ecstasy without the tension release of explosive orgasm. You're so filled with kundalini that it streams continuously of its own accord throughout your body. The intense sensations are more like pulsing electromagnetic waves than just a few physical spasms. You feel those same ecstatic vibrations that normally come from a jewel explosion, but you feel them everywhere.

You've undoubtedly experienced an energy orgasm if you've trembled, shivered, felt hot flashes, or had goose bumps all over. The electricity makes your nerves twitter, the magnetism makes your muscles quiver, and the erotic charge makes your body shake.

Wouldn't you love to spend more time sizzling, crying out, and undulating with pleasure? And making your sweetheart thrash madly, flail wildly, and shriek uncontrollably?

Orgasmic Sensations

It's kundalini that propels you to both physical and energy orgasms. They both trigger similar sensations. But physical ones are limited to what you get for the few seconds of muscle tension release and male ejaculation. Energy orgasms, on the other hand, can grow stronger and stronger and go on and on.

Instead of being localized in your jewels, an energy orgasm feels like geysers of erotic electricity flood you, grip you, and milk you all over. Streaming orgasmic energy makes you swoon and undulate. Surging showers of ecstasy make your entire biofield pulse in time with your beating heart.

The fiery sensations engulf you as if every cell climaxes. You feel lighter and lighter, like floating away on a cloud of pleasure.

Somraj was surprised by his first energy orgasm. Suddenly, he was hot and tingly all over. His feet felt like throbbing vajras. His head was on fire. His body was undulating and jackknifing, shaking wildly. He thought he must have screamed because his throat was sore afterward. It was just like those intense spasms of pleasure during ejaculation. But he wasn't coming wetly while the surge of ecstasy played on and on.

Energy orgasms create sexual fireworks inside your body. Five main things happen while you implode: electrical discharges, detonations, fire, waves, and vibrations.

Sexual electricity shows up as rays, bolts, sheets, and streamers of sexual energy. It can spark, sizzle, crackle, streak, and zap. It can even give you a shock. When the charge isn't very strong, it can feel like a buzzing current flowing through your circuits.

Kundalini detonating inside feels like bursts, blasts, and bangs. The pyrotechnics start as a gleam or sparkle and grow into a blossom or eruption. Sexual fire can produce tendrils of heat, flames, and fireballs. When mellow, it's more like smoldering embers or hot coals. The behavior of kundalini closely resembles moving water like lapping waves or tidal surges. It can feel like it's seeping, pooling, cascading, or fountaining.

Spreading kundalini doesn't always follow a steady process like water heating up before it boils. Sometimes it's more like diffusion, the creeping heat gradually filling you up. Diffusion is what happens when you pour a few drops of strong, dark coffee into a glass of water.

Vibrations like trembling muscles or spasming jewels is the last category of sexual energy manifestations. Kriyas, which jolt your tissues, can grow into swaying, shimmying, and shuddering. They start with a twitch, shiver, or tremor and can grow into continuous streaming.

Implosion

Energy orgasms are *implosive* instead of explosive. Instead of releasing vitality with a big bang, the kundalini reverberates internally. Since you contain the sexual energy without fighting it, it's recycled.

Imploding energy is the ultimate pathway to multiple and full-body orgasms. Because you're not resisting the buildup of erotic charge, it expands, flooding your pleasure balloon and energy channels. Kundalini spreads out of your jewels, energizes all your chakras, and recirculates throughout your whole body. The implosion feels more like rolling thunder than a sharp clap of lightning.

Sometimes the first physical responses that accompany an implosive orgasm are quiet and slow. Other times the outbursts of liquid fire throw you around.

Enjoying energy orgasms is how you harness the full power of kundalini to fill your whole body with orgasmic bliss. It's a vastly different experience than the physical release of tension that most lovers experience.

How to Implode

You'll limit your energy orgasms if your inner flute and other channels aren't free-flowing. If parts of your body are armored or there are blocks between your chakras, the subtle energy won't be able to expand and reach these less alive tissues.

If the onslaught of so much power makes you uncomfortable, you'll fight the impending tsunami. The more complete your surrender, the less resistance your kundalini will encounter when it begins to implode. Which is why your success with implosive energy orgasms rests on how well you practice the Tantric attitude and the five cornerstones of ecstasy.

Of course, you have to fill your pleasure balloon with enough fuel to implode. Everything you've read about so far—loveplay, strokes, schemes, sweet spots, sweet rhythms, hot links, peaks, plateaus, passion circuits, energy circles—is how you prepare your kundalini to implode.

Running and streaming energy is key. Instead of restricting your excitement to the small, confined area around your jewels, draw the electrical stream upward through your inner flute and encourage it to all parts of your body.

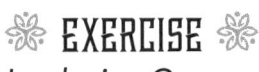

EXERCISE
Implosive Orgasm

1. Try this exercise solo at first.
2. Consciously run energy upward to charge all your chakras.
3. Enjoy a long, slow buildup of pleasure with multiple peaks.
4. It helps if you occasionally level and float for a moment after each peak. As the voltage of your repeated peaks increases, the sensations will become more intense.
5. Instead of letting the top blow off in explosive orgasm, extend the peaks into plateaus.
6. When the excitement threatens to make you tense up or lose control, use orgasmic breathing to spread the kundalini. Slow and deepen your breathing. Let out low, guttural sounds that vibrate your jewels or other chakras.
7. To intensify your experience, totally focus on every little microsensation.

It helps if you concentrate on the tidal waves of energy caressing your mind, body, and spirit. Picture the energy rippling through you as surges, pulses, or sparklers. Imagine it's a blinding white light filling your body, the whole room, or the whole planet. Visualize that you're ascending on updrafts, soaring high above the earth, floating on billowy clouds, or orbiting in weightless space.

As your biofield fills with more kundalini, you'll feel more and more pleasure. At some point the kundalini experience takes over of its own accord, blooming and streaming inside. The key here is to surrender to the electromagnetic waves imploding throughout your body.

You can learn to set off implosions without physically stimulating your erogenous zones. But energy orgasms triggered during jewel union are our favorites.

Full-Body Orgasm

Most lovers experience orgasm localized in the jewels. In contrast, a full-body orgasm spreads everywhere. Since it's caused by channeling sexual energy out of the jewels, it's an implosive orgasm that spreads orgasmic sensations everywhere.

Jeffre remembers a powerful experience that led to a full-body orgasm. It started when she had a series of short, sharp peaks. Each time she felt a delightful surge of sensation spreading out from her jewels. At first it felt like streamers of sexual charge filling her central channel.

Then, the peaks started to rise and spread into longer plateaus. As her pleasure balloon expanded, the streamers morphed into billiard balls of titillation shooting up from her jewels.

After a few of these cycles, the streamers blossomed out of her inner flute making her sizzle and shake all over. By relaxing and surrendering, the shivers spread through her, culminating in involuntary spontaneous kriyas.

The plateaus launched her into a Valley of pleasure where her body vibrated in response to the spreading spasms of sensation. It wasn't a steady state of erotic high but rather a shifting kaleidoscope. Sometimes she floated in a trancelike state of ecstasy. Other times pleasure grenades detonated with a rising rush of chills, heat flushes, and goose bumps. They felt like an inner mushroom cloud making her scalp erotically tingle.

The different surges of orgasmic sensations were like electrical discharges deep in her pelvis. The expanding shock waves of pleasure rippled out of her G-crest in all directions. As the rising surges filled her physical and energy body, she quivered, quaked, and shook all over.

That's a perfect snapshot of a full-body orgasm: the orgasmic contractions sweeping through, first vibrating here, then there, then everywhere.

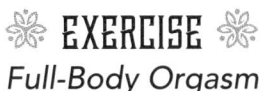

EXERCISE
Full-Body Orgasm

This practice is similar to the Implosive Orgasm Exercise but focuses more on spreading the energy all over.

1. Try this exercise solo at first.
2. As you charge your chakras, concentrate on spreading the kundalini to your feet, hands, head, and everywhere else.

3. Enjoy a long, slow buildup of pleasure with multiple peaks.
4. When the excitement threatens to make you tense up or lose control, use orgasmic breathing to spread the kundalini throughout your body. Slow and deepen your breathing. Let out low, guttural sounds that vibrate your jewels or other chakras.
5. To intensify your experience, totally focus on every little microsensation.

Summary and Action Steps

- An energy orgasm is a plateau of ecstasy without the tension release of explosive orgasm.
- Imploding energy is the key to multiple orgasms.
- To implode, run energy up your inner flute to charge all your chakras.
- Learn to bypass explosive orgasm with the Implosive Orgasm Exercise.
- Enjoy the sexual fireworks that energy orgasms create inside your body.
- Practice spreading kundalini to implode everywhere with the Full-Body Orgasm Exercise.

Chapter 24
IN ORBIT

Have you ever felt you were outside your physical body, filling the whole room, the whole house, the whole universe? When you circle kundalini back and forth at multiple points, your pleasure balloons expand to fill your biofields.

Chakra to chakra passion circuits catalyze energy exchange between lovers. When you connect two or more of your chakras with your lover's, you naturally interchange more kundalini. That's when the strongest energy exchange happens. Then your energy fields spread across the space you share and merge, oscillating with sexual electromagnetism.

When you both feel a deeper, wider, more powerful pulsing, you fully open yourselves to each other. And when you connect your bodies, minds, and spirits, your boundaries disappear.

The sharing of biofields, which figure 22 on page 230 shows, has the power to transform your and your lover's consciousness. You can use this soul merger to go beyond space and time, beyond the outside world as you know it. This is how you can fuse your body, mind, and soul with your lover's.

When you hook up passion circuits and energy circles as we described in PART 6, Kundalini Currents, you open your inner self to a deeper outpouring of love. It allows you to connect with your partner at multiple levels of heart, mind, and soul.

A sense of wonder engulfs you both. You're consumed with the rapture of divine union with your beloved. It feels as if time stops. You lose touch with the outside world for a moment as you soar far above the material plane.

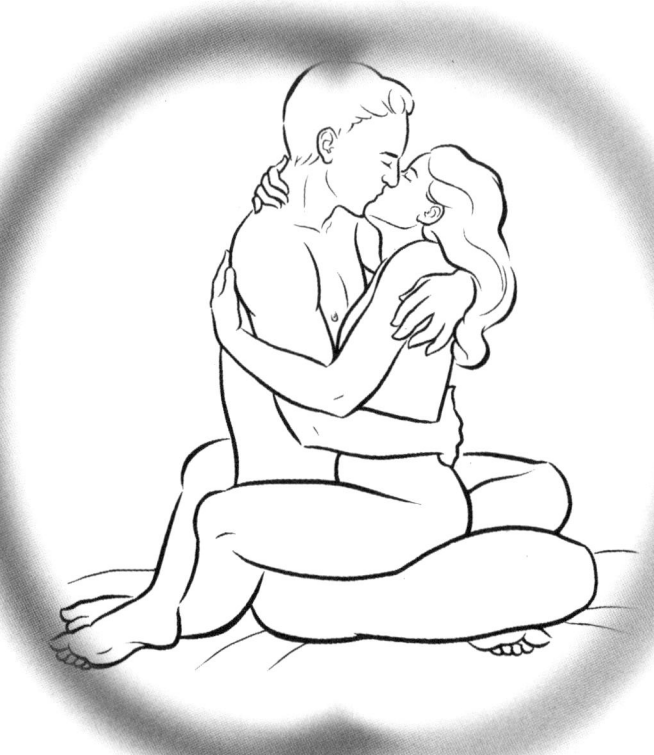

Figure 22: Merged Biofields

It feels like you're both catapulted beyond the atmosphere into orbit at the edge of outer space. This level of joint ecstasy is an altered state of consciousness, a portal into a trance of non-ordinary reality, like that achieved through dreaming, meditation, or psychedelics.

To understand orbiting together, we're going to share how to expand your orgasmic state into a lofty plane and merge yourselves into one.

Extended Orgasm

Masters and Johnson measured explosive orgasms in the range of four to twelve seconds. With the energy practices of Supernatural Sex, you'll be able to extend your energy orgasms much longer.

Extended orgasms are high plateaus of excitement that last longer and feel more ecstatic than short bursts of energy. Instead of throwing off the electrical charge, conserving it can extend them for thirty seconds, sixty seconds, or many minutes.

You can extend your orgasms either physically or energetically. The physical approach requires that you keep stimulating aroused sweet spots. You do this in spite of the fact that, on the downslope of the pleasure peak, your body's level of arousal will drop.

Here's how to practice extending your orgasms. You may want to practice this exercise solo first using your hands or sex toys before jewel union.

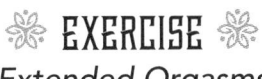
EXERCISE
Extended Orgasms

1. Agree the partner who orgasms first will carry on.
2. Giver, maintain the stimulation right through the trough after orgasm.
3. If necessary, pause momentarily and slow your strokes until the receiver's arousal ascends again.
4. Receiver, even though your heartbeat, breathing, and blood pressure cool off a bit, keep actively reaching for more pleasure.

This takes some dedication since sweet spots, notably clios and vajra heads, become ultrasensitive after an explosive climax. But if you keep at it, you can trigger orgasm after orgasm, which can gradually morph into an extended physical orgasm.

The energetic path to extended orgasm begins by running energy to peak after peak. First, you'll experience single implosive climaxes, the male version without ejaculation. When you repeat this cycle several times, the rising peaks will gradually merge into longer, higher plateaus. The intense excitement of streaming kundalini will trigger extended energy orgasms.

If you flow with it, your level of pleasure will climb higher and higher, reaching amazing states of ecstasy.

The O-Zone

A series of extended energy orgasms can create high plateaus of excitement that persist. These plateaus can coalesce into a continuous state of ecstasy. We call this the *orgasmic zone*, or O-Zone for short.

The O-Zone is a self-sustaining state of passion where strong tides of kundalini stream through you. It requires little or no effort for the continuous vibrations and slow contractions to surge for minutes. You can float in the O-Zone on and off for hours with little or no further sexual stimulation. As the plateaus extend, the ecstasy becomes so intense that it feels like an endless climax.

Not only does soaring in the O-Zone feel awesome, but it's good for you. Afterward you feel less irritable, less stressed, happier, and healthier. In the O-Zone, your consciousness expands while your heart rate and blood pressure go down.

Floating in the O-Zone is why Supernatural Sex is often described as *meditative sex*. You've been there if you've ever

- stayed aroused after sex for up to twenty-four hours,
- been able to restart those earth-shaking orgasmic sensations just by recall, or
- been so high that you never wanted the sexual ecstasy to end.

Entering the O-Zone is like sinking into an ocean of rapture and letting go.

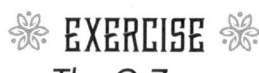

EXERCISE
The O-Zone

1. When you find yourself floating in a high plateau of ecstasy while making love, just let go.
2. Relax in the high state of arousal.
3. Go with the flow and let the currents carry you.
4. Surrender to the rising tide of ecstasy and let yourself be transported somewhere else.

While it's true that being able to enter the O-Zone at will is a special skill, when you do, it feels like something magical is happening to you. The continuous orgasmic waves of supreme bliss take you and you float in the timeless, transcendent void.

Non-Ordinary Reality

Have you ever been so mesmerized during sex that you found yourself in a delightful trance or euphoric reverie?

In the O-Zone, your body becomes an empty sieve to some otherworldly lifeforce passing through you. You feel wide-open at the top to the cosmic forces of the sky, and at the bottom to the bosom of the earth. You're transformed into an open channel for the communion between body and soul, physical and spiritual, human and Divine. You feel overwhelmed by a sensation of being "breathed by the universe."

The O-Zone is a timeless place beyond thought, beyond agendas, beyond separation. Your mind drifts, your body feels weightless, and your soul soars. You feel like you're floating somewhere else, separate from mundane reality.

Without effort, you're buoyed up by the ecstasy that bubbles up of its own accord. As you become more in tune with the vital energy that animates your body, you'll arrive in a space where you know that bliss is your native state.

Riding the wave of ecstasy up to the O-Zone launches you into an altered state of consciousness. In the continuous orgasm space, you're transported into a non-ordinary reality. This takes you into an altered dimension outside normal space. Your ego quiets, your continuously chattering monkey-mind stills, and your spirit is transfixed. It seems as if time stands still.

Neuroscientists have recently explained why this happens.[25] Rhythmic stimulation alters brain activity. If neurons are excited multiple times in quick succession, they're focused in a way that's hypnotizing. That makes you block out everything else except the intense sensations.

To access non-ordinary reality, stop the world by fully experiencing the moment. Attend to the rich sensory input available in each subsequent now, but without much thinking. Or, more simply put, immerse yourself fully in the Tantric attitude.

---

25. Amanda Monteiro. "Neuroscientist Explains How Orgasms Can Be Used to Reach an 'Altered State' of Consciousness." Collective-Evolution.com. 9/26/2017. https://www.collective-evolution.com/2017/09/26/neuroscientist-explains-how-orgasms-can-be-uses-to-reach-an-altered-state-of-consciousness/.

Orbiting

In the non-ordinary reality of the O-Zone, something supernatural happens. Synchronized energy orgasms catapult you up to a persistent plateau where you're overwhelmed with an intense flood of euphoric sensations. You ascend past the stratosphere into a higher orbit.

Floating in orbit together becomes a sacred energy event, an intimate unity, and a bonding of lifeforces separate and distinct from momentary tension release. When you're lucky, you find yourself levitated into the oneness of spiritual communion with the entire universe.

When you soar in orbit, the erotic charge keeps flowing of its own accord. In this elevated playing field, it's amazing how much you feel because your bodies are more sensitive and more receptive. Your sensory field opens to a wider spectrum of sensations. And the impact of those sensations is dramatically magnified. More cells awaken and vibrate, sending off their own sparklers of sexual electricity.

To get the idea, imagine you look through a telescope at one spot on the moon. Then, all at once, your vision widens to cover the whole disk. And that happens to your sense of touch, smell, taste, and hearing at the same time. It's like going from black and white to color. Like jumping from two dimensions to three. Like flying where you once walked.

It's the continuous streaming of sexual passion that shoots you into orbit. Because the current is steady, you don't have to work at it. Any touch, lick, or stroke seems to detonate ecstasy grenades like splashes in a still lake. And without anything in the way, they keep rebounding.

Every bit of arousal is amplified. The sexual electromagnetism floods you and between you. But since there's little resistance, the surface of the pond remains still while the current below gets stronger.

Oneness

In orbit, there's a kind of spiritual communion between lovers that we call *oneness*. Oneness is the deepest form of connection between hearts, minds, and spirits. It's a phenomenon of consciousness where you transcend individual bodies, chattering minds, and independent egos. You feel as if you and the cosmos are one. It's an unlimited, timeless, altered state of spiritual communion with each other and the entire universe.

The barriers between you dissolve when your biofields merge as we showed previously in figure 22 on page 230. Any sense of separation disappears. You can't tell where your body ends, and your beloved's body begins. The whole concept of "you" and "me" makes no sense when your souls merge into one.

This is the driving force behind Tantric lovers who devote themselves fully to making love through all chakras at once. This is the essence of sacred sex.

To reach for it, focus on extending your plateaus, creating passion circuits, and opening energy circles. Envision drawing kundalini from each other's jewels. Visualize a connection at each chakra. Move the energy up your inner flutes synchronously to your crown chakras. Send it out the top of your head into your beloved's crown, creating a psychic energy circle.

When the kundalini streaming through both of you vibrates at the same frequency, the dividing lines between your physical forms disintegrate. It's as if you are one being with one body. Then your union of love feels divine, your spiritual communion feels total.

In these glimpses of a higher dimension, you enter a timeless void and feel one with all of existence.

Summary and Action Steps

- To make your physical orgasms last longer, use the Extended Orgasms Exercise.
- Let your high plateaus of ecstasy merge into the O-Zone, where you seemingly float forever.
- Practice entering the state of continuous orgasm with the O-Zone Exercise.
- Immerse yourself in the Tantric attitude to access non-ordinary reality.
- Allow the continuous streaming of sexual passion to shoot you into orbit.
- Sacred sex, when you make love through all chakras at once, energizes a sense of oneness.

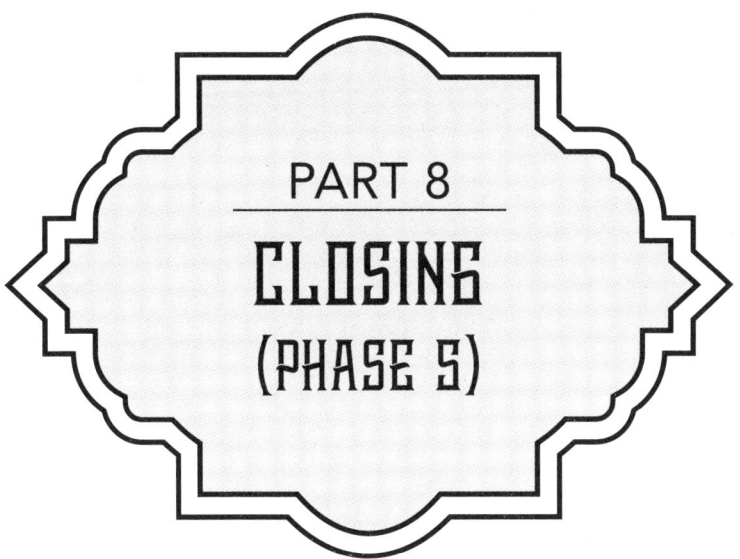

PART 8
CLOSING (PHASE 5)

In this last part, which consists of chapter 25, we'll summarize the journey this book has taken you through. The following chapter emphasizes what to do in phase 5 to wrap up your sacred sexual encounters. The Conclusion and Final Sentiments that follow stress how to keep your energetic connection alive and well.

You must realize that our purpose has been much more than sharing a few bullet points. Since it's our last chance, we want to encourage you to practice. Any kind of sex, and especially Supernatural Sex, isn't transformed into ecstatic bonding overnight. We hope you signed up for the long haul and regularly experiment with the exercises we've suggested. That's the essence of Tantra and most useful spiritual paths: to transform your life, you need to put these concepts into action.

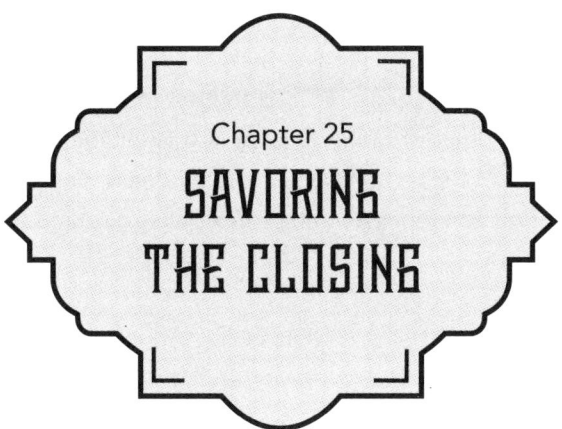

Chapter 25
SAVORING THE CLOSING

After you've cavorted in the Valley at length and climbed to the O-Zone, you'll eventually enter the Closing phase of Supernatural Sex, phase 5. That's where you wind down and wrap up.

After you've come together, make a point of coming down together with love and consciousness. It's important, at least for a few minutes of the Closing phase, to remain as connected as you were while making love. Wrapping up your time together should be a sweet, intimate bonding passage where you appreciate what you've shared, relate your experience with each other, or just hold one another.

Afterplay

Basking in the afterglow extends your pleasure and deepens your intimacy. Because Supernatural Sex is a marathon and not a sprint, coming down should also be a slow and sensual affair. Just when your energy channels are most intertwined, you don't want to break them abruptly.

Women's bodies—and those of sensitive men—stay aroused long after lovemaking winds down. Continuing physical contact with gentle caresses and melting hugs feels good and cements your energetic bond. Whether one or both of you have enjoyed an explosive release or not, you've generated and exchanged lots of energy.

Kundalini will still be alive within you. The intense physical exertions that dramatically exercised your body need time to gradually subside as your metabolism returns to normal. Orgasmic energy still streams, sensations still wash your insides, and electromagnetic currents still sweep through your nervous system. And between you.

Your altered state will persist, at least temporarily. Somraj still remembers his first lovemaking demonstration in front of a large Tantra workshop where he vibrated afterward for an hour while coming down. Being with it, relaxing into it, surrendering into it helped him ground, integrate, and extend the transformation.

Savor

Don't rush off. Take a moment to savor what you feel without hurrying on to something else. Lie still and feel. Breathe slowly and deeply. Notice what your body experiences now. Relish the tastes, smells, and sights of each other. Appreciate the peaceful, relaxing sensations. Relax in meditation if that works for you.

As the fires of passion subside, do whatever you can to extend the warm glow that's suffusing you. Women especially experience some of the most beautiful emotions and sensations while bathed in the afterglow of intense kundalini exchange.

Maintain the harmony you've cocreated with tenderness, consideration, and compassion. Lingering together is better than turning over and falling asleep. Make it a point to stay connected instead of suddenly jumping up. If you abruptly break your physical connection, the shock of disconnecting all your passion circuits and energy circles can be jarring.

Closing is a wonderful time for some sweet, long, melting cuddling and snuggling. Actively show your love and affection. Lying together and spooning keeps the exchange of warmth and energy alive between your aligned chakras. Slowly and gently massage each other or just stay still holding each other. Share some kisses that seal your bond.

Disconnecting your jewels slowly and tenderly is most appreciated, especially when the earth moved and you're still shivering and quaking. A vital reason to avoid abrupt separation after jewel union is that you've merged your biofields. It may take up to twenty minutes before your energy bodies can be lovingly pried apart.

We like to keep Somraj's vajra inside as long as possible. The natural process of his organ contracting and easing its way out minimizes the jarring shock that sudden withdrawal could cause. Of course, if you've worn a condom, you'll want to make sure it doesn't come off inside. Once you slip out is the perfect time to honor your safe sex agreements and tie off the open end.

Closure

Once you can move, create energetic closure by sitting across from each other. Do a heart bonding with your eyes locked together and your hands over each other's chest. This is the simplest yet most poignant closing ceremony because it draws energy up into your hearts and exchanges it.

Or you can place one hand on your beloved's jewels and the other over their chest in a heart bonding. You may or may not want to speak at this point.

Do whatever you can to stay energetically linked when you begin moving. Feed each other with finger foods and share some wine or fresh water. One of our favorite things to do once we get up is to bathe or shower together, washing each other's jewels.

If you're able to be verbal, share what you've experienced and what's going on inside you. The Closing phase is the perfect time to express gratitude, appreciation, and celebration.

Exchange sweet everythings. Maybe you want to share what was new, special, or different for you. Maybe you want to mention what gave you the most pleasure and what you most enjoyed doing to your playmate. Laughing together is a great way to express your joy and thanks for the things that only your love could have brought.

We understand that talking sometimes feels right as you wind down, but not other times. If you're willing, a great way to get closure about what you started is by revisiting the original partnering questions.

Were your desires satisfied? Were your concerns addressed? Were your boundaries respected?

If you've been practicing some of the exercises in this book, exchanging feedback about your sexual experience can help you both build on what you learn. You may want to ask some specific questions about how your honey reacted at certain times. And you might want to mention how you reacted at different points in your escapade.

What do you want more of or less of next time? What did you learn or get confused about? What would you like to learn more of? And though a little mental connection is great, don't overdo talking right now. You don't want to suddenly get yanked out of your settling body into your head.

That's the spirit of the Closing phase, keeping the love and joy you've shared alive as long as you can.

Summary and Action Steps

- Stay connected physically and energetically during the Closing phase.
- Take your time to bask in the afterglow together.
- Create closure with a heart bonding, exchange sweet everythings, and share your experience.

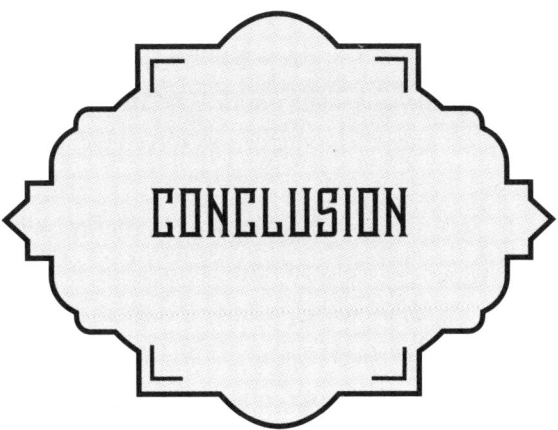

CONCLUSION

Supernatural Sex is an extraordinary style of sexual union. This holistic approach to Tantric sex doesn't just focus on orgasm, but creates a continuously orgasmic, altered state of the shared ecstasy of love. While the spiritual consciousness and energy tools we related may seem mystical to the average lover, it's not really magic.

Summary of the Pathways

The following is a reminder of the pathways to Supernatural Sex that we have been discussing throughout the book.

- **Chakras:** Make love at all chakras to open multiple heart, mind, and soul energy channels while you give and receive pleasure.
- **Partnership:** Empower men, women, and same-sex lovers as partners to expand intimacy, sensuality, and pleasure.
- **Jewel Union:** Thoroughly understand the mechanics of jewel union to build erotic charge and exchange sexual electricity.
- **Kundalini:** Run and stream kundalini, the universal lifeforce energy that surges through and between you, at will.
- **Sweet Spots:** Find and trigger all twenty male and thirty female sweet spots.
- **The Valley:** Extend your play in the Valley by surfing peaks and extending plateaus.

- **Pleasure Balloon:** Using sweet spots, sweet rhythms, and hot links, pump energy into your pleasure balloon to fill your biofield.
- **Orgasms:** Develop mastery over orgasms so that you can choose when and what type you enjoy, including dry, wet, blended, extended, full-body, and simultaneous ones.
- **Stamina:** Make love longer with extended sexual stamina for men and women.
- **Share:** Exchange kundalini using passion circuits and energy circles to feel and share each other's ecstasy.
- **Energy Orgasm:** Instead of exploding, implode with all the sensations of physical orgasm and recycle kundalini without depleting sexual energy.
- **In Orbit:** Reach high plateaus of ecstasy with repeated energy orgasms until they merge into the O-Zone and catapult you into orbit.
- **Oneness:** Lose any separation and totally merge with your beloved and the entire universe as you journey on the pathway to divine communion.

Final Sentiments

We've been exploring and following these pathways to Supernatural Sex for more than twenty years. As a result, lovemaking has never been dull, boring, or routine. It keeps getting better and we keep learning new things about ourselves and each other. In spite of all the normal stresses most people experience with work, health, stress, and relationships, our all-chakra connection keeps our love alive.

Reading this book and starting on this path makes us all part of one big tribe. So we hope to hear of your progress, problems, and questions using the contact information on page 245.

We hope you can develop your sex life into your own unique style. We hope we've achieved our aim of showing you something different and better than ordinary sex. May your every erotic encounter become supernatural. And may your life be transformed into everything you've ever dreamed of.

Love,
Somraj and Jeffre

Contact Us

We look forward to hearing from you with your successes, problems, revelations, questions, and feedback. Contact us at Somraj@Supernatural.Sex or visit us at tantraattahoe.com.

BIBLIOGRAPHY

Anand, Margot. *The Art of Sexual Ecstasy*. Los Angeles: Tarcher, 1989.

Barbach, Lonnie, PhD. *For Yourself*. New York: Penguin, 1976.

Bodansky, Steve, PhD, and Vera Bodansky, PhD. *The Illustrated Guide to Extended Massive Orgasm*. Alameda, CA: Hunter House, 2002.

Bonheim, Jalaja. *Aphrodite's Daughters*. New York: Fireside, 1997.

Borelli, Lizette. "The Sex Moves Women Want: Clitoral Stimulation Helps Female Orgasm, Study Finds." *Newsweek*, September 21, 2017. https://www.newsweek.com/sex-moves-female-orgasm-relationships-dating-669154.

Brauer, Alan P., MD, and Donna J. Brauer. *ESO*. New York: Warner, 1983.

Carrellas, Barbara. *Urban Tantra*. San Francisco: Celestial Arts, 2007.

Castleman, Michael. *Great Sex*. New York: Rodale, 2004.

Chang, Jolan. *The Tao of Love and Sex*. New York: Penguin Books, 1977.

Chia, Mantak, and Manccwan Chia. *Cultivating Female Sexual Energy*. Huntington, NY: Healing Tao Books, 1986.

Chöpel, Gedün. *Tibetan Arts of Love*. Translated by Jeffrey Hopkins. Ithaca, NY: Snow Lion Publications, 1992.

Chu, Valentin. *The Yin-Yang Butterfly*. New York: Tarcher/Putnam, 1993.

Danielou, Alain. *The Complete Kama Sutra*. Translated by Alain Danielou. Rochester, VT: Park Street Press, 1994.

Deida, David. *The Enlightened Sex Manual: Sexual Skills for the Superior Lover.* Louisville, CO: Sounds True, 2007.

Doniger, Wendy, and Sudhir Kakar. *Kamasutra.* New York: Oxford University Press, 2002.

Douglas, Nik. *Spiritual Sex.* New York: Pocket Books, 1997.

Douglas, Nik, and Penny Slinger. *Sexual Secrets.* Rochester, VT: Destiny Books, 2000.

Douglass, Marcia, PhD, and Lisa Douglass, PhD. *The Sex You Want.* New York: Marlowe, 1997.

Easton, Dossie, and Catherine A. Liszt. *The Ethical Slut.* San Francisco: Greenery Press, 1997.

Garrison, Omar. *TANTRA: The Yoga of Sex.* New York: Causeway, 1964.

Goddard, Jamie, and Kurt Brungardt. *Lesbian Sex Secrets for Men.* New York: Plume/Penguin, 2000.

Hirschlag, Ally. "Why Some Women Orgasm Easier Than Others." *SheKnows*, May 6, 2016. https://www.sheknows.com/love-and-sex/articles/1120927/why-some-women-have-better-orgasms.

Joannides, Paul. *Guide to Getting It On!* Waldport, OR: Goofy Foot Press, 2000.

Ladas, Alice Kahn, Beverly Whipple, and John. D. Perry. *The G Spot and Other Discoveries about Human Sexuality.* New York: Dell, 1982.

Long, Barry. *Making Love: Sexual Love the Divine Way.* Sydney: Barry Long Books, 2006.

Monteiro, Amanda. "Neuroscientist Explains How Orgasms Can Be Used to Reach an 'Altered State' of Consciousness." *Collective-Evolution*, September 26, 2017. https://www.collective-evolution.com/2017/09/26/neuroscientist-explains-how-orgasms-can-be-uses-to-reach-an-altered-state-of-consciousness/.

Morin, Jack, PhD. *Anal Pleasure and Health.* San Francisco: Down There Press, 1998.

Muir, Charles, and Caroline Muir. *Tantra The Art of Conscious Loving.* San Francisco: Mercury House, 1989.

Mumford, Dr. Jonn. *Ecstasy Through Tantra.* St. Paul, MN: Llewellyn Publications, 1975.

Odier, Daniel. *Desire: The Tantric Path to Awakening*. Rochester, VT: Inner Traditions/Bear, 2001.

———. *Tantric Quest: An Encounter with Absolute Love*. Rochester, VT: Inner Traditions/Bear, 1997.

Osho. *TANTRA: The Supreme Understanding*. Pune: The Rebel Publishing House, 1991.

———. *The Tantra Experience*. Shaftesbury, UK: Element, 1994.

———. *Tantra Spirituality and Sex*. Pune: Osho International, 1983.

Pokras, Somraj. *Male Multiple Orgasm*. Berkeley, CA: Amorata/Ulysses, 2007.

Pokras, Somraj, and Dr. Jeffre TallTrees. *Female Ejaculation*. Berkeley, CA: Amorata/Ulysses, 2009.

Ramsdale, David, and Ellen Ramsdale. *Sexual Energy Ecstasy*. New York: Bantam, 1985.

Reich, Wilhelm. *The Function of the Orgasm*. New York: Noonday Press, 1973.

Richardson, Diana. *The Heart of Tantric Sex*. Alresford, UK: O Books, 2003.

Riley, Kerry, with Diane Riley. *Tantric Secrets for Men*. Rochester, VT: Destiny Books, 2002.

Schwartz, Dr. Bob, and Leah Schwartz. *The One Hour Orgasm*. Houston: Breaththru Publishing, 1995.

Streicher, Lauren, MD. "Science Says Yes to Female Ejaculation." *EverydayHealth*. August 25, 2016. https://www.everydayhealth.com/columns/lauren-streicher-midlife-menopause-and-beyond/female-ejaculation/.

Sundahl, Deborah. *Female Ejaculation and the G-Spot*. Alamed, CA: Hunter House, 2003.

Tunneshende, Merilyn. *Don Juan and the Art of Sexual Energy*. Rochester, VT: Bear, 2001.

Van Lysebeth, André. *TANTRA The Cult of the Feminine*. York Beach, ME: Samuel Weiser, 1995.

Wikoff, Johanina, PhD, and Deborah S. Romaine. *The Complete Idiot's Guide to the Kama Sutra*. Indianapolis: Alpha Books, 2000.

Winks, Cathy, and Anne Semans. *The Good Vibrations Guide to Sex*. San Francisco: Cleis Press, 1994.

Winston, Sheri. *Women's Anatomy of Arousal*. Kingston, NY: Mango Garden Press. 2010.

Zilbergeld, Bernie, PhD. *The New Male Sexuality*. New York: Bantam, 1992.

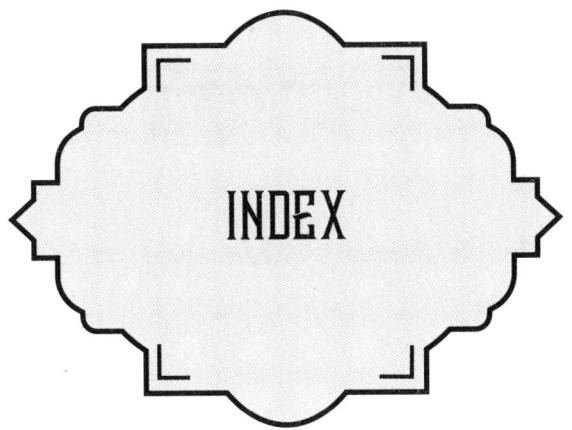

INDEX

5 Ss, 202, 205, 209

A-Spot, 67, 121, 146, 151, 195, 196
Aftershocks, 220–222
Afterplay, 239
Albolene, 49
Alcohol, 27
All-Chakra Lovemaking, 103
Altered State, 1, 4, 13, 23, 126, 137, 148, 230, 233, 234, 240, 243
Alternate Peaking, 206, 207
Amrita, 69, 218
Anal Canal, 56, 57, 64, 127–129, 152
Anal Cushion, 128
Anal (Rosetta) Sex, 23, 25, 99, 125, 126, 130–133, 135, 136, 194, 208
Anal Toy, 130
Anatomy, 2, 3, 6, 14, 53, 59, 68, 74, 82, 127, 194
Anus, 43, 56, 125, 141
Arabia/Arabian/Arabic, 5, 13, 93, 153
Armoring, 99, 106, 126, 128, 135, 138, 139, 141, 142, 164, 176, 187, 225

Arnold Kegel, MD, 94
Arousal, 3, 5–7, 23, 27, 39, 43, 45, 46, 49, 51, 56, 64, 66, 68, 69, 74, 76, 82, 87, 89, 94, 123, 135, 138, 148, 157, 163, 168, 174, 201, 203, 206, 207, 213, 214, 218, 231, 232, 234, 239
Asana, 119

Backdoor, 57, 126–129, 131–133, 135, 141, 195
Balance, 7, 21, 37, 50, 119, 135, 143, 159, 160, 166, 167, 185, 206
Bartholin's Glands, 49, 62, 69
Base (Vajra's Base), 54, 55, 57, 107, 108, 194–196
Be in Your Body, 27, 28, 145
Beginner's Mind, 26, 31, 176, 206
Big O, 23, 28, 77, 145, 149, 155, 202, 221
Biofield/Bio-energetic Field, 17, 21, 45, 75–78, 96, 146, 173, 174, 177, 179–181, 197, 207, 224, 226, 229, 230, 235, 240, 244

Biochemicals, 57, 75, 174
Bioelectric, 43, 76, 174, 191
Bladder, 55, 57, 65–67, 218
Blended Orgasm, 213, 219, 220, 222
Bliss, 19, 23, 25, 87, 213, 225, 232, 233
Blockage, 137, 175–177, 181
Blossoms, 19, 22, 75, 146, 181, 184, 188, 195, 206, 224, 227
Body Armoring, 126, 138, 142, 176
Body Gate, 128, 176
Body Honoring, 28, 33
Body Language, 38, 162, 163, 169
Boner, 53
Boundary, 37, 38, 40, 168, 169, 229, 241
Brain, 33, 45, 49, 83, 156, 174, 179, 180, 184, 233
Brinkmanship, 145, 148
Bulb (Vajra's Bulb), 56
Bulbocavernosus Muscle, 61, 216
Bulbospongiosus Muscle, 61
Butt Plug, 130, 194

Canal, 56, 57, 59, 63–69, 111, 121, 125, 127–129, 135, 140, 152
Cannabis, 27
Carl Jung, 12, 160
Cervix, 67, 69, 70, 121, 140, 146, 151, 194, 196
Chakra, 21, 22, 41, 46, 48, 71, 74, 76, 79–83, 85, 88, 90, 95–97, 120, 138, 154, 155, 173, 175–177, 179, 180, 183, 189, 193, 194, 196, 198, 208, 219, 220, 225–229, 235, 240, 243
Chakra Breathing, 80, 82, 85, 176

Channel, 3, 7, 8, 21–23, 27, 36, 38, 56, 76, 77, 79, 83, 85, 87, 90, 95, 103, 109, 126, 137–139, 142, 145, 162, 167, 171, 173–179, 181, 183, 184, 191, 193, 195–198, 202, 206, 211, 219, 221, 225, 227, 233, 239, 243
Check In, 39–41, 103, 133, 135, 163
Chemistry, 2, 5, 11, 43
China/Chinese, 5, 13, 73, 109
Churn, 104, 152, 158
Circumcised, 53, 54
Clearing, 83, 88, 97, 121, 135, 137–142, 164, 176, 214
Climax, 8, 13, 19, 23, 28, 32, 57, 75, 77, 96, 161, 178, 206, 211, 213–216, 218–220, 222, 224, 231, 232
Climbing, 6–8, 22–24, 76, 145, 147, 149, 211, 231, 239
Climbing Phase, 7, 22, 24, 211
Clio, 62–66, 68–70, 104, 119, 122, 123, 134, 151, 152, 161, 162, 164, 192–197, 215, 216, 221, 231
Cliogasm, 216–218, 221
Clitoris/Clitoral, 19, 62, 122, 216
Closing Phase, 8, 237, 239, 241, 242
Closure/Closing, 6–8, 22, 23, 176, 237, 239–242
Communication, 13, 31, 35–41, 102, 120, 123, 126, 132, 139, 148, 159, 161, 164, 198, 220
Communication Tools, 39, 40
Communion, 2, 137, 233–235, 244
Concentration, 51, 56, 77, 127, 128, 146, 147, 149, 153, 167, 192, 195, 202, 226, 227

Concerns, 14, 37, 38, 40, 131, 169, 241
Condom, 37, 50, 104, 129, 130, 134, 135, 241
Conduit, 79, 83, 184
Conscious Breathing, 26, 30, 33, 89, 176
Consciousness, 1, 2, 12, 13, 19, 23, 26, 27, 47, 73, 88, 138, 148, 178, 229, 230, 232–234, 239, 243
Consent, 11, 25, 31, 37, 45, 168
Contraction, 23, 36, 76, 93, 94, 105, 214, 217, 220, 221, 227, 232
Convulsion, 16
Cornerstone, 87–91, 93–97, 111, 148, 160, 162, 173, 174, 178, 180, 188, 203, 206, 225
Corona, 54
Corpse Posture, 27, 33
Corpus, 63
Coupling, 7, 8, 111, 155, 178, 191, 194, 204, 207
Cowgirl, 114
Crest, 204–206
Crotch, 23, 174
Crown, 47, 54, 62, 80, 83, 96, 107, 108, 152, 179, 180, 196, 235
Crura, 63, 122, 151
Cues, 103, 106, 108, 148, 162, 164
Cuff, 68–70, 105, 106, 111, 215
Cul-de-Sac, 67, 121, 146, 151, 195, 196
Current, 1, 7, 19, 21, 71, 75, 79, 140, 148, 171, 173, 174, 176–178, 180, 183, 184, 186, 187, 195, 196, 198, 208, 211, 224, 229, 232, 234, 240

Cycle/Cycling, 22, 145, 155, 157, 158, 163, 171, 198, 203–205, 207, 209, 214, 225, 227, 231, 244

Dancing on the Verge, 147–149
De-armoring, 176, 181
Desire, 2, 4, 12–14, 17, 25, 30, 31, 33, 35, 37, 38, 40, 41, 46, 48, 64, 75, 82, 103, 161, 162, 169, 191, 203, 218, 241
Diana Richardson, 107
Diffusion, 224
Digits, 194
Digital Play, 193, 198
Dildo, 67, 70, 121, 194
Divine, 1–4, 12, 15, 16, 23, 28, 33, 40, 43, 53, 77, 83, 95, 137, 156, 160, 179, 208, 229, 233, 235, 244
Doggie Style, 115
Dominant, 36, 126, 161, 167, 192
Dominate/Domination, 35, 48, 102, 119, 125, 126, 159, 167–170
Dry Orgasm, 178, 214, 215, 221

Ecstasy, 1, 3, 5, 7, 12, 14, 15, 19, 21, 25, 27, 33, 36, 40, 53, 71, 76, 82, 83, 87, 88, 90, 94, 95, 97, 111, 125, 126, 139–141, 145, 148, 159, 162, 163, 167, 171, 173–175, 178–181, 184–188, 203, 208, 211, 217, 223–225, 227, 228, 230–235, 237, 243, 244
Edging, 145, 148, 149
Ejaculate/Ejaculation, 57, 66, 67, 69, 94, 101–103, 149, 176, 187, 201,

204, 214, 215, 217–221, 223, 224, 231
Electricity Generators, 183
Electricity, 1, 2, 4, 5, 7, 14, 15, 19, 21, 23, 45, 47, 73–76, 79, 80, 95, 104, 105, 108, 140, 147, 148, 171, 173, 180, 181, 183–185, 187, 189, 196, 197, 201, 209, 211, 223, 224, 226, 227, 231, 234, 243
Electromagnetism, 14, 185, 229, 234
Empower, 3, 5, 35, 103, 105, 243
Energy Circle, 22, 171, 192, 197–199, 201, 203, 206, 211, 220, 226, 229, 235, 240, 244
Energy Orgasm, 4, 8, 19, 21, 23, 38, 76, 178, 186, 187, 221, 223–226, 228, 230–232, 234, 244
Energetic Clearing, 137, 176
Engorged, 49, 57, 64, 66, 68, 69, 101, 105, 121, 174
Equal Relations, 110
Erect/Erection, 5, 22, 26, 40, 46, 49, 53–58, 60, 62–68, 70, 77, 94, 101, 103, 104, 107, 110, 111, 122, 125, 135, 140, 151–153, 162, 183, 198, 204, 214, 218
Ernst Gräfenberg, MD, 65
Erogenous Zone, 2, 7, 8, 19, 31, 43, 46–48, 53, 55, 57–59, 62, 64, 65, 67, 68, 123, 126, 134, 151, 155, 162, 193, 194, 196, 198, 220, 226
Erotic Charge, 4, 5, 46, 89, 95, 146, 168, 171, 174, 175, 179, 185, 186, 191, 195, 197, 206, 223, 225, 234, 243
Erotic Movement, 88, 91, 97, 173
Exchange, 1, 3, 7, 16, 22, 23, 36, 37, 40, 48, 74, 96, 120, 135, 149, 167, 168, 170, 171, 195, 196, 199, 206, 207, 229, 239–244
Excite, 1, 5–8, 11, 15, 19, 21–23, 27, 29, 36, 38, 45, 49, 57, 62, 68, 69, 75, 87, 89, 103, 109, 119, 123, 147, 149, 151–153, 157–159, 163, 168, 169, 171, 175, 177–179, 184, 185, 187, 189, 193, 194, 198, 201, 203, 204, 207–209, 214, 216, 218, 226, 228, 231–233
Explode, 6, 14, 15, 17, 21, 23, 53, 62, 75, 77, 109, 156, 166, 176, 178, 187, 202, 208, 213, 214, 217–221, 223, 225, 226, 228, 230, 231, 239
Explosive Orgasm, 6, 15, 21, 62, 176, 178, 202, 213, 214, 221, 223, 226, 228, 230
Extended Orgasm, 3, 230, 231, 235
Eye-Gazing, 30, 83, 191, 197

Fantasy, 30, 35, 39, 48, 159, 162, 168–170
Feedback, 38–41, 131, 133, 159, 162–164, 191, 241, 245
Female Ejaculation/Female Ejaculate, 66, 69, 217, 218, 221
Female Orgasm, 122, 215, 216, 218, 222
Finger, 38, 39, 41, 45, 47, 48, 54, 58, 61, 64, 66, 67, 103, 105, 107, 108,

125, 128–131, 133, 135, 139, 140, 142, 164, 165, 177, 179, 180, 183, 193, 194, 202, 204, 208, 213–215, 241

Fire, 1, 4, 15, 19, 75, 83, 89, 91, 95, 147, 179, 180, 184, 188, 209, 224, 225, 240

Fireworks, 3, 19, 87, 146, 181, 184, 185, 195, 224, 228

First Thrusts, 106, 111, 126, 131, 133, 134, 168

Five Cornerstones of Ecstasy, 87, 95, 111, 148, 162, 173, 174, 178, 180, 188, 203, 225

Flare, 68, 197

Flow, 2, 7, 15, 19, 22, 23, 27, 36, 39, 45–47, 57, 73, 74, 79, 82, 83, 85, 87, 88, 90, 94, 95, 102, 108, 119, 138, 140, 146, 148, 149, 154, 155, 157, 161, 163, 167, 168, 171, 173–177, 180, 183–188, 191, 192, 197, 198, 201, 203, 204, 206, 208, 211, 219–221, 224, 225, 231, 232, 234

Flow Principle, 180

Foreskin, 53, 54, 58, 108

Fornix, 67, 70, 121

Fourchette, 61, 68, 152, 196

Frenulum, 54, 152

Full-Body Orgasm, 77, 173, 177, 179, 184, 186, 198, 225, 227, 228

G-Crest, 66, 68–70, 119, 121, 125, 135, 136, 140, 146, 151, 152, 154, 164, 166, 193–196, 217, 218, 227

G-Crest Rub, 154

G-Spot, 19, 22, 57, 65, 135, 136, 152, 164, 195, 214, 215, 221

G-Spot Orgasm, 214, 215, 221

GI/Gastrointestinal, 56, 57, 60, 127, 129

Giver, 5, 16, 28, 47, 126, 131–133, 138–142, 159, 161–164, 166, 193, 197, 206, 219, 231

Glans, 54, 62

Goals, 5, 11, 24, 25, 28, 29, 33, 88, 130, 131, 145, 155, 218

Gradual Insertion Method, 130, 136

Groin, 15, 28, 49, 184

Habituate/Habituation, 155, 157, 158, 208

Hand, 12, 14, 19, 22, 31, 41, 46–48, 55, 58, 62, 79, 83, 93, 103, 107, 108, 120–122, 130, 134, 165, 176, 179, 180, 184, 187, 188, 193–195, 197, 198, 202, 213, 221, 224, 227, 231, 241

Hand-Assist, 103, 104, 107, 134, 152, 193

Hard On, 55, 103

Healing, 5, 7, 33, 137, 138, 140–142

Heart, 1–3, 12, 14, 22–24, 27, 29, 30, 32–34, 37, 40, 41, 45, 46, 48, 68, 74, 77, 80, 83, 95, 96, 105, 107, 120, 161, 165, 174, 177, 179, 181, 191, 197, 198, 213, 215, 224, 229, 232, 234, 241–243

Heart Bonding, 40, 241, 242

Heart-Centered, 191

Heart Meditation, 30, 34
Heat, 14, 15, 28, 37, 40, 45, 74, 75, 95, 106, 140, 146, 180, 181, 183, 184, 196, 197, 224, 227
High Union, 110, 120
Hindu, 12, 13
Hood, 62, 63, 68, 69, 122
Hormones, 11, 23, 37, 43, 45, 46, 68, 137, 162, 174, 213
Hot Link, 7, 22, 171, 175, 191–195, 197–199, 201, 203, 215, 216, 219, 220, 226, 244
Houston's Valves, 129, 135

Implode/Implosion, 224–226, 228, 244
Implosive Orgasm, 209, 225–228
India/Indian, 2, 5, 12, 13, 21, 40, 47, 73, 79, 109
Initial Entry, 6, 7, 22, 99, 101–104, 107, 108, 133, 143, 151, 153, 154, 164, 167, 193, 196–198
Initial Entry Cues, 103
Inner Flute, 83–85, 87, 93–95, 148, 175, 176, 178–181, 197, 203, 208, 225–228, 235
Inner Lips, 59–62, 64, 65, 68, 69, 122, 196
Inner Sphincter, 128, 134, 135, 152
Inner Yoni, 50, 59, 61, 63–70, 151, 216
Intercourse, 2, 5, 7, 8, 29, 138
Intimacy/Intimate, 2–4, 7, 8, 13, 21, 25, 29, 30, 33, 34, 38, 41, 46, 51, 76, 77, 120, 126, 162, 175, 179, 191, 217, 218, 221, 234, 239, 243
Introitus, 61

Jewel, 5, 7, 8, 13, 15, 16, 19, 21–23, 29, 31, 36, 38, 43, 45–49, 51, 53, 54, 62, 64, 68, 73–77, 82, 90, 91, 93, 95, 99, 101–103, 105, 106, 108–110, 119, 120, 122, 123, 131, 134, 137–139, 141, 143, 146, 147, 152, 153, 155, 157, 159, 164, 165, 167, 168, 171, 173, 174, 176–180, 183–189, 191–199, 202, 204, 208, 213, 216, 217, 219–221, 223–228, 231, 235, 240, 241, 243
Jewel Size, 106, 109, 123, 152
Jewel Union, 5, 7, 8, 22, 29, 36, 45, 49, 51, 68, 74–77, 91, 99, 101, 102, 106, 109, 119, 120, 122, 123, 131, 134, 138, 141, 143, 146, 153, 157, 159, 167, 171, 179, 188, 191–195, 197–199, 204, 208, 216, 219, 220, 226, 231, 240, 243
Juice, 45, 95, 148, 180

Kaleidoscopic Rhythm, 15, 154–156, 158
Kama Sutra, 13, 21, 47, 48, 53, 109, 110, 152, 193
Karezza, 153, 157, 204
Kegel, 94–97, 221
Kink/Kinky, 39, 109, 156, 157, 168, 194
Kissing, 1, 48, 74, 120, 193, 195, 197, 198, 240

Kriya, 91, 204, 208, 225, 227
Kundalini, 1–4, 7, 8, 17–19, 21, 22, 24, 27, 32, 36–38, 43, 46, 53, 71, 73–79, 83, 85, 88–91, 95, 96, 102, 105, 109, 119, 120, 125, 126, 135, 137, 138, 142, 143, 145, 149, 152, 153, 155, 157, 163, 168, 171, 173–181, 185–189, 191, 195–199, 202–204, 207, 208, 211, 217–221, 223–229, 231, 232, 235, 239, 240, 243, 244

Labeling, 164, 170
Labia, 59, 60
Labia Majora, 59
Labia Minora, 60
Last Stroke Technique, 29, 33, 133
Lava Lamping, 149
Lead/Leader/Leadership, 16, 35–37, 41, 62, 67, 104, 105, 132, 139, 152, 156, 160, 161, 164–169, 198, 204, 219
Leapfrogging, 206, 207
Legs (Clio's Legs), 63, 64, 68, 69, 122, 151, 195, 196
Levitate, 23, 185, 234
LGBTQIA, 3
Libido, 3, 17, 46, 79, 137, 203
Lifeforce, 1, 3, 7, 12, 14, 17, 19, 21, 73, 75–77, 79, 80, 83, 95, 139, 149, 156, 174–176, 180, 184, 186, 198, 202, 208, 233, 234, 243
Lips, 22, 32, 45, 47, 59–62, 64, 65, 68–70, 104, 105, 119, 122, 193, 194, 196
Lip Furrow, 60

Loosening Your Body, 187–189
Love Sounds, 87, 90, 91, 95–97, 173, 178, 202
Lovemaking, 1, 2, 7, 16, 28, 29, 41, 82, 83, 90, 97, 99, 103, 120, 126, 132, 142, 148, 152, 155–158, 168, 189, 191, 193, 198, 201, 204, 219, 239, 240, 244
Loveplay, 6, 7, 22, 43, 45, 46, 48, 49, 51, 60, 74, 101, 103, 107, 111, 132–134, 137, 142, 143, 153, 154, 167, 195, 198, 213, 225
Low Union, 111
Lower Sponge, 64, 66, 68–70, 121, 125, 146, 151, 195, 196
Lube/Lubricant, 41, 49–51, 104, 107, 129, 131, 133–135, 161, 194
Lubrication, 31, 49, 58, 62, 64, 67, 69, 126, 129, 217
Lust, 11, 25, 38, 74, 75, 80, 82

Magnetism, 14, 21, 43, 80, 168, 184, 186, 223
Male G-Spot, 215
Male Orgasm, 125, 214, 215, 221
Man-Above Position, 112, 119–122, 131, 194
Man-Kneeling Position, 113, 120–122, 131, 194
Margot Anand, 25, 40, 53, 73, 83, 94, 97, 139, 141, 167, 185
Massage, 21, 31, 47–49, 51, 82, 93, 103, 104, 122, 133, 138, 139, 142, 147, 151, 181, 193, 194, 197, 203, 240

Masturbation, 31, 141
Meatus, 54
Meditate / Meditation / Meditative, 2, 4, 12–14, 24, 26, 30, 33, 34, 46, 73, 80, 82, 83, 85, 88, 153, 156, 157, 176, 180, 191, 219, 230, 232, 240
Meditative Sex, 232
Menopause, 46, 49, 62, 137, 176
Metabolism, 45, 68, 203, 213, 214, 239
Mind's Eye, 88, 94, 175, 180
Mindfulness, 2, 13, 26, 74
Missionary, 36, 107, 112
Monitor / Monitoring, 31, 102, 159, 163, 164, 166, 168, 206
Mons / Mons Pubis, 59, 62
Mound of Venus, 59, 62
Multiple Orgasm, 37, 218, 219, 228

Nadi, 79, 83, 85, 175, 191
Namastés, 40
Nerves / Nerve Endings / Nervous System, 1, 14, 19, 21, 27, 45, 47, 54, 56, 62, 64, 66, 68, 69, 73, 79, 90, 91, 125, 127, 128, 138, 147, 151, 165, 174, 175, 184, 186, 203, 207, 209, 223, 240
Nipple, 22, 32, 46–48, 68, 193
Nonverbal Communication, 38, 133, 161, 162, 164, 198

O-Zone (Orgasmic Zone), 211, 232–235, 239, 244
Oneness, 23, 234, 235, 244
Open-Ended Question, 39–41

Oral Sex, 7, 36, 39, 50, 193, 197
Orbit, 8, 211, 226, 229, 230, 234, 235, 244
Ordinary Sex, 2–4, 11, 12, 16, 35, 75, 82, 244
Orgasm / Orgasmic, 1–8, 11, 12, 14, 15, 17, 19, 21, 23, 24, 31, 33, 35, 37, 38, 57, 58, 62, 64, 65, 67–69, 71, 74, 76–79, 82, 83, 87, 88, 91, 93–97, 103, 104, 119, 122, 125, 137, 138, 140, 145, 147–149, 153, 155, 156, 159, 171, 173–180, 184–187, 191, 193, 197, 198, 201, 202, 204, 205, 207–209, 211, 213–228, 230–235, 239, 243, 244
Orgasm Gap, 12, 103
Orgasmic Breathing, 95–97, 104, 140, 148, 176, 178–180, 185, 191, 202, 208, 226, 228
Orgasmic Energy, 7, 17, 74, 78, 82, 93, 147, 149, 153, 155, 171, 186, 201, 204, 207, 208, 224, 239
Orgasmic Surfing, 204
Osmolality, 50
Outer Lips, 59, 60, 68
Outlet, 54, 55, 61, 65, 104, 122, 146, 151, 194, 196, 216
Outer Sphincter, 128, 134

P-Spot, 56, 214, 215
Pain / Painful, 31, 46, 62, 101, 108, 111, 119, 126, 128, 133, 138–141, 159, 164, 169, 175, 176
Partner Peaking, 205, 207, 209

Partner/Partnering/Partnership, 3, 4, 7, 9, 11, 13, 16, 26, 28, 30, 35–41, 46, 58, 62, 68, 70, 74, 80, 90, 91, 97, 101–104, 107, 119, 126, 130–134, 136, 139, 140, 143, 145, 151, 154, 156, 159, 161–171, 177, 191, 194, 196, 197, 205–207, 209, 213, 215, 218, 220, 229, 231, 241, 243

Partnering Questions, 37–40, 46, 74, 80, 90, 102, 107, 130–132, 134, 140, 145, 154, 156, 161–163, 168, 169, 191, 207, 241

Passion Circuit, 7, 22, 191, 192, 195–199, 201, 203, 206, 211, 220, 226, 229, 235, 240, 244

Pathway, 2–9, 11, 79, 82, 83, 126, 128, 137, 148, 173, 175, 185, 186, 188, 220, 225, 243, 244

Peaking Cycle, 203–205, 207, 209

Pearl (Clio's), 62, 63, 68, 69, 122, 162, 193, 194

Pelvic Floor, 57, 58, 67, 80, 92–94, 96, 111, 138, 178, 185, 187, 214

Pelvic Rocking, 91, 95, 96

Pelvis/Pelvic, 21, 23, 46, 57–59, 63, 67, 69, 80, 83, 91–97, 107, 108, 111, 120, 121, 132, 138, 141, 146, 151, 165, 166, 178, 185, 187, 204, 213–217, 227

Penis (see Vajra), 5, 22, 43, 53, 110, 121

Penis Extender, 121

Penetrate/Penetration, 7, 8, 14, 22, 53, 71, 99, 101–103, 105, 107, 108, 110, 111, 119, 121, 125, 126, 128, 129, 131, 133–136, 141, 152, 162, 186, 194, 195

Perineum, 55, 56, 58, 60, 64, 68, 104, 180, 214

Permission, 33, 104, 108, 131, 133, 134, 136, 163, 164

Physical Orgasm, 24, 213, 214, 220, 231, 235, 244

Plateau/Plateauing, 6, 7, 21, 96, 201, 205, 207–209, 211, 219, 220, 223, 226–228, 231, 232, 234, 235, 243, 244

Pleasure Balloon, 20, 21, 23, 37, 71, 75–78, 83, 87, 96, 146–149, 157, 159, 163, 173, 176–181, 184, 185, 187, 189, 197, 201, 202, 205, 207, 215, 218, 219, 223, 225, 227, 229, 244

Plexus/Plexi, 66, 69, 70, 121, 151, 196

Pocket Rocket, 194

Pompoir, 93, 111, 168, 195, 196

Porn, 48, 119

Postillionage, 194

Pre-come, 58

Premature Ejaculation, 94, 102, 103, 149, 187

Premature Penetration, 101, 108

Probe, 50, 106, 129, 194

Prostate Gland, 56–58, 125, 135, 214, 221

Pubic Bone, 59, 63, 66, 67, 93, 121, 122

Pubic Grinding, 122, 123, 151

Pubococcygeal Muscles, 93

Puffy Cuff, 68–70, 105, 215

Quickie, 11, 13, 37, 55, 111

Raising Kundalini, 77, 171, 179–181
Rear-Entry Position, 115, 119–121, 131, 152, 194
Receiver, 5, 16, 28, 47, 73, 74, 91, 126, 131–133, 139–142, 152, 159, 161, 162, 164, 166, 170, 174, 181, 186, 193, 197, 206, 219, 231
Rectum, 57, 64, 66, 126, 127, 129, 130, 135
Resistance, 99, 135, 175, 176, 225, 234
Resolution, 6, 7
Resonance/Resonant, 188, 196
Responsibility, 5, 17, 25, 30, 31, 34–38, 79, 82, 102, 103, 119, 130, 162
Responsive/Responsiveness, 61, 66, 101, 159, 163, 169, 206
Reverse Cowgirl, 114
Reverse Kundalini, 176
Role-Play, 48, 159, 168–170
Rosetta, 23, 25, 29, 32, 39, 43, 49, 55, 56, 58, 60, 64, 67, 74, 93, 99, 101, 102, 125–137, 141, 142, 152, 162, 164, 165, 176, 186, 193–197, 208, 214, 215
Rosetta Clearing, 137, 141, 142, 176
Rosetta Entry, 133, 134, 136
Run/Running Energy, 22, 91, 137, 155, 173, 177–179, 181, 183, 191, 196, 220, 226, 228, 231

Sacred Sex, 6, 32, 235
Sacred Space, 40, 41, 46, 74, 80, 130, 191, 215
Safe word, 169
Same-Sex, 99, 111, 168, 243
Scheme, 143, 146, 151, 153–155, 158, 159, 164, 167, 203, 225
Scrotum, 22, 32, 55, 56, 58, 134, 194, 197
Self-Pleasure, 31, 32, 34, 49, 70, 90, 137, 176, 178, 185, 202, 203, 208, 215, 218
Semen, 55, 58, 178, 214, 218
Sensate Focus, 28, 33
Sex Flush, 1, 28, 46, 68, 103, 165, 227
Sex Toy, 13, 31, 48, 64, 121, 130, 179, 194, 202, 214, 231
Sex-Negative, 137, 142
Sex-Positive, 5, 25, 137, 142, 215
Sexology/Sexologists, 5, 21, 55, 66, 67, 215, 217
Sexual Energy, 1, 2, 8, 9, 12–15, 17, 21, 25, 27, 37, 47, 73–75, 79, 80, 87, 93, 94, 108, 109, 138, 145, 149, 153, 168, 171, 173, 174, 176–178, 181, 183, 184, 188, 189, 201, 202, 213, 224, 225, 227, 244
Sexual Position, 7, 53, 107, 109, 111, 120, 121, 168, 191, 194, 198, 202, 205
Sexual Posture, 13, 111, 119, 120, 123, 131, 157, 194, 195
Sexually Transmitted Disease (STD), 50, 129
Shakti, 12, 160, 161, 166, 167
Sheri Winston, 68, 74
Shiva, 12, 160, 161, 166, 167
Shiva-Shakti Game, 167, 170

Short Cycles, 157, 158, 203
Side-to-Side Position, 116, 119–121, 131, 152
Sigmund Freud, MD, 138, 160
Simultaneous Peaking, 206
Simultaneous Orgasm, 213, 219, 222
Sitting Position, 117, 120, 121, 132, 152, 194
Soft Entry, 107, 108
Solo Peaking, 203, 209
Soul, 2–4, 12, 14, 15, 22, 24, 34, 37, 41, 46, 74, 76, 77, 80, 83, 87, 88, 155, 229, 233, 235, 243
Spasm, 14–16, 58, 91, 93, 103, 126, 165, 186, 188, 195, 197, 213–215, 223–225, 227
Sphincter, 55, 56, 61, 64, 126–128, 130, 134, 135, 152, 196, 213, 214, 216
Spine, 17, 46, 57, 73, 80, 93, 177, 179
Spirit/Spiritual, 1–4, 6, 11–13, 16, 22, 23, 25, 30, 32, 33, 43, 45, 80, 88, 120, 125, 135, 156, 174, 178, 179, 209, 215, 226, 229, 233–235, 237, 242, 243
Spongy Cylinders, 55, 58
Stamina, 94, 244
Standing Position, 118–121, 132, 152, 194
Stimulate/Stimulation/Stimuli, 2, 6, 7, 17, 27, 43, 45, 46, 48, 49, 51, 53, 55–57, 62–65, 70, 73, 87, 90, 110, 119, 121–123, 134, 135, 138, 151, 152, 155, 158, 162, 167, 186, 188, 191, 193, 194, 198, 203, 205, 208, 214–221, 226, 231–233

Stream/Streaming Energy, 71, 83, 185, 194, 205, 226
Strokes, 1, 7, 15, 28, 29, 32, 33, 36, 39, 48, 60, 61, 66, 68, 69, 91, 103, 105–108, 119, 121, 122, 129, 133–135, 143, 146, 147, 151–159, 164–167, 179, 186, 193–196, 202–205, 208, 209, 216, 218, 221, 225, 231, 234
Submissive/Submit/Submission, 35, 36, 119, 125, 126, 168–170
Subtle, 1, 14, 17, 19, 21, 22, 27, 38, 47, 73, 75, 79, 82, 83, 108, 133, 148, 149, 153, 155, 164, 165, 173, 174, 176, 186, 221, 225
Supernatural Sex, 2–9, 11–14, 16, 17, 19, 21–28, 30, 31, 35–38, 40, 41, 43, 45, 46, 75, 77, 80, 83, 87, 90, 99, 103, 104, 107, 109, 120, 137, 143, 145, 151, 156, 157, 159, 161, 163, 165–167, 171, 173, 178, 195, 196, 205, 206, 213, 215, 230, 232, 234, 237, 239, 243–245
Surf/Surfing, 7, 147, 171, 204, 205, 207, 209, 211, 218, 223, 243
Surfing Peaks, 204, 205, 209, 243
Surrender, 14, 15, 28–30, 83, 135, 161, 162, 167, 177, 203, 208, 219, 225–227, 232, 240
Sweet Everythings, 39–41, 74, 83, 120, 133, 241, 242
Sweet Rhythm, 7, 21, 102, 143, 146, 147, 153, 156–159, 164, 186, 201–204, 206, 226, 244
Sweet Spot, 7, 8, 19, 21, 22, 24, 43, 47, 53–62, 64, 66, 67, 70, 71, 74–77,

83, 95, 109, 119–123, 125, 138, 143, 146, 147, 151–153, 155, 156, 158, 159, 163, 164, 167, 186, 191, 194–199, 201–203, 213–217, 219–221, 231, 243, 244

Swoon, 153, 186, 196, 224

Sync/Synchronize, 39–41, 96, 97, 159, 166, 170, 171, 205, 207, 234, 235

Taboo, 126, 168

Tantra/Tantric, 1–9, 11–13, 17, 19, 22, 23, 25, 26, 28, 30–32, 46, 47, 51, 66, 73, 74, 76, 80, 82, 87–91, 95–97, 102, 107, 130, 133, 137, 139–141, 145, 153, 155, 158–160, 163, 173, 176, 177, 183, 186, 188, 201, 215, 217, 223, 225, 233, 235, 237, 240, 243

Tantric Attitude, 9, 25, 26, 28, 30–32, 46, 47, 74, 76, 80, 88–90, 102, 130, 133, 139, 145, 155, 158, 159, 163, 176, 183, 215, 225, 233, 235

Tantric Breath, 87, 89–91, 95–97, 173

Tantric Touch, 47, 51, 82

Taoism/Taoist, 13, 21, 153, 204

Taoist Nines, 153, 204

Tenting, 69

Testicles, 49, 55, 56, 58, 194

Thigh Grooves, 60

Third Eye, 48, 80, 88, 179, 181, 198

Thrusts, 1, 15, 21, 29, 67, 69, 90, 91, 102, 105, 106, 108, 111, 121, 122, 126, 131, 133, 134, 143, 146, 151–154, 156, 158, 159, 161, 162, 165, 168, 193–196, 203, 204, 221

Thumbgasm, 193

Tongue, 61, 64, 156, 194

Trigger, 21, 31, 45, 57, 64, 65, 67, 77, 102, 156, 163, 197, 199, 206, 214–222, 224, 226, 231, 243

Tumescent/Tumescence, 49, 55, 68

Turn-On/Turned-On, 1, 5, 7, 11, 17, 21, 27, 30, 32, 36, 45, 46, 48, 49, 88, 90, 91, 97, 106, 119, 120, 132, 134, 137, 152, 154, 156, 157, 159, 162–164, 166, 169, 175, 176, 184, 185, 187, 191, 197, 201, 204, 206, 209, 215, 217

Uncircumcised, 58, 108

Unequal Relations, 110

Upward Energy Draw, 179

Urethra, 55, 61, 65, 66, 70, 121, 151, 214, 216, 218

Urethral Sponge, 65, 66, 70, 121, 218

Uterus, 66, 69, 217

Vagina/Vaginal, 5, 22, 43, 50, 59, 61, 62, 64, 67, 110, 125, 129, 166

Vajra, 5, 22, 29, 31, 35, 36, 39, 40, 43, 49, 53–55, 57, 58, 62, 64, 67–69, 74, 77, 90, 93, 101–105, 107–111, 119–122, 125, 128, 132–135, 138, 140, 141, 146, 147, 151–154, 156, 159, 161, 164–168, 186, 193–198, 213, 214, 216, 221, 224, 231, 240

Vajra Yoni-Massage, 104, 107, 108, 193, 196

Valley, 6–8, 22–24, 75, 135, 143, 145–147, 149, 197, 201, 206, 207, 211, 227, 239, 243
Vasocongestion, 46, 58, 69
Verbal Communication, 38, 133, 198, 241
Verge, 21, 145, 147–149, 223
Vestibular Bulbs/V-Bulbs, 64, 68, 69, 122, 151, 195, 196
Vestibule, 61, 62, 64, 68, 104, 152
Vibrator, 119, 122, 164, 194
Visualize/Visualization, 21, 47, 75, 85, 88, 94–97, 139, 142, 156, 173, 174, 177, 178, 180, 181, 185, 186, 188, 197, 198, 226, 235
Voice, 25, 32, 80, 87, 90, 91, 105, 157, 179, 188, 202
Voltage, 23, 149, 184, 185, 189, 207, 211, 226
Vulva, 5, 43, 59

Wave, 4, 14–16, 19, 23, 75, 101, 125, 141, 145, 147, 157, 159, 163, 175, 185, 187, 206, 208, 209, 213, 216, 217, 221, 223, 224, 226, 227, 232, 233
Wet, 14, 16, 47–50, 56, 74, 105, 139, 142, 146, 163, 165, 174, 183, 193, 198, 214, 217, 224, 244
Wilhelm Reich, MD, 138
Woman-Above Position, 114, 120, 121, 132
Womb, 66, 67, 69, 151, 176, 215, 216

Yab-Yum, 117, 194, 198
Yes-No Question, 39, 41
Yin and Yang, 159–161, 167, 177
Yoga, 27, 73, 91, 97, 119, 187
Yoni, 5, 22, 29, 32, 36, 39, 43, 49, 50, 53, 59–70, 74, 77, 93, 99, 101–111, 119, 121–123, 125, 126, 128, 129, 132–135, 137–142, 146, 151–153, 156, 162, 164–166, 168, 176, 186, 192–198, 215–218, 221
Yoni Clearing, 121, 138–141
Yoni Erection, 68, 70, 218
Yonigasm, 216–218, 221

To Write to the Authors

If you wish to contact the authors or would like more information about this book, please write to the authors via their personal email, **Somraj@Supernatural.Sex**, or in care of Llewellyn Worldwide Ltd. Both the authors and the publisher appreciate hearing from you and learning of your enjoyment of this book and how it has helped you. Llewellyn Worldwide Ltd. cannot guarantee that every letter written to the author can be answered, but all will be forwarded. Please write to:

Somraj Pokras and Jeffre TallTrees, PhD
Somraj@Supernatural.Sex
℅ Llewellyn Worldwide
2143 Wooddale Drive
Woodbury, MN 55125-2989

Please enclose a self-addressed stamped envelope for reply,
or $1.00 to cover costs. If outside the U.S.A., enclose
an international postal reply coupon.

Many of Llewellyn's authors have websites with additional information and resources. For more information, please visit our website at http://www.llewellyn.com.

GET MORE AT LLEWELLYN.COM

Visit us online to browse hundreds of our books and decks, plus sign up to receive our e-newsletters and exclusive online offers.

- Free tarot readings • Spell-a-Day • Moon phases
- Recipes, spells, and tips • Blogs • Encyclopedia
- Author interviews, articles, and upcoming events

GET SOCIAL WITH LLEWELLYN

Find us on 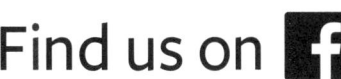 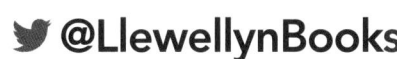 @LlewellynBooks

www.Facebook.com/LlewellynBooks

GET BOOKS AT LLEWELLYN

LLEWELLYN ORDERING INFORMATION

 Order online: Visit our website at www.llewellyn.com to select your books and place an order on our secure server.

 Order by phone:
- Call toll free within the US at 1-877-NEW-WRLD (1-877-639-9753)
- We accept VISA, MasterCard, American Express, and Discover.

 Order by mail:
Send the full price of your order (MN residents add 6.875% sales tax) in US funds plus postage and handling to: Llewellyn Worldwide, 2143 Wooddale Drive, Woodbury, MN 55125-2989

POSTAGE AND HANDLING

STANDARD (US):(Please allow 12 business days)
$30.00 and under, add $6.00.
$30.01 and over, FREE SHIPPING.

CANADA:
We cannot ship to Canada, please shop your local bookstore or Amazon Canada.

INTERNATIONAL:
Customers pay the actual shipping cost to the final destination, which includes tracking information.

Visit us online for more shipping options.
Prices subject to change.

FREE CATALOG!

To order, call
1-877-NEW-WRLD
ext. 8236
or visit our website

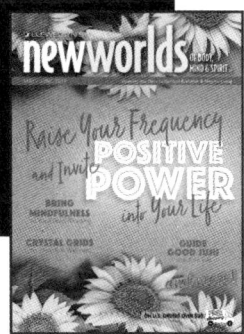